CONTAGIOUS MADNESS

Karen Kellock Ph.D.

Manual for Superior Men

This is a complete theory based on Einstein physics,
Political Psychology, Systems Theory
and Archetypal Psychiatry.

FORMULA

All success attraction
All disease obstruction
All recovery elimination

You must fast on all three

OBSTRUCTIONS:

People
Habit
Food

CONTAGIOUS MADNESS

They didn't treat you as special, unique, talented or significant.   You're treated with indifference/love was conditional. They compared you to others like you're fullabull. Early rejection explains the insane drive for greatness and the survival panic leading to suicide. The world imposes BS then weak friends create a mess blocking success.   Significance is a child of God and that gives you purpose, no more seen as odd.

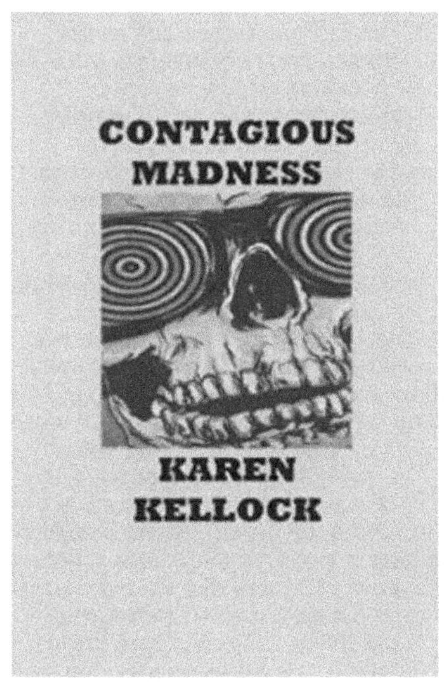

SEEN AS SCUM

THE WICKED FLIP-FLOP
GOD SEES WHO YOU WILL BE
CREEPS WORM THEIR WAY IN
IMPOSTOR SYNDROME
CHRISTIAN DIVAS?
JEALOUS OF YOUR BLESSINGS
BREAKING DOWN THRU HUMILIATION
HUMILIATION OF DECEPTION
OBEYING A BAD MAN IS SATAN
JEALOUS SUPERIORS AND FRIENDS
HE KNOWS WHAT HE IS DOING
TRIGGERING YOU CONSTANTLY
EMOTIONAL IMMATURITY
THE RENAISSANCE MAN IS GONE
CALLOUSNESS OF YOUTH
DIS-FATTEN: SUPERFLUOUS THOUGHTS
NEW AGE NERDS ESTABLISHMENT
TRIGGERING SELF-ESTEEM LEAKS
EMOTIONAL VIOLENCE
DECEPTION IS EMOTIONAL VIOLENCE
SILENCE IS HELLISH
SILENCE IS A RUDDER OF CONTROL
CHAOS FROM EMOTIONAL VIOLENCE
SAVIOR ARCHETYPE BEGINS AS LOWEST ASS
CHAOS MAKERS ARE EMOTIONALLY VIOLENT
CHAOS CREATES SOUL TIES
INVALIDATION IS VIOLENCE
BLAME-SHIFTING IS VIOLENCE
VIOLENCE OF DISACKNOWLEDGEMENT
OLDER IS OUTA TURMOIL AND TORTURE
PLAYING VICTIM IS THE MODERN CURSE
MISJUDGEMENT BY INFERIORS
LIBERALS THINK ALL ARE GOOD
CLOWNS ARE RUNNING THE CIRCUS
"BE LIKE US, THE GOOD PEOPLE"
WOMEN SHOULD STUDY MEN
MEN BOND IN PURSUIT

SEEN AS SCUM

CONTAGIOUS MADNESS

TRAUMA AND BOUNDARIES
NASTY PROJECTIONS
SELF-SERVING FAMILY MYTHS
NEGLECT CREATES MENTAL ILLNESS
BRAIN-SHRINK FROM SHUN-STINK
AGEIST NEGLECT STARTS EARLY
FORGIVE OR HATE YOURSELF
BAD MOM ARCHETYPE
NOTHINGNESS: ON TOP OF WORLD
REPENTANCE AND THE PINK CLOUD
LETHAL MENTAL DISORDERS
THE DEMON IS AN UGLY GREEN THING
THE RESULTS ARE GOOD *AND* BAD
YOU'RE A PERSON NOT A DISEASE
CARNIVORE VS LOWFAT REVERSALS
TWO-SPEED FOOD LIFE
CONTRADICTIONS AND REVERSALS
OBSTRUCTIONS & THE CREATIVE ACT
AUDIT NETWORK
IMAGINARY GOOD IS BORING
A MONUMENTAL ACHIEVEMENT: YOU
AS BODY RECEDES BRAIN EXPANDS
PEOPLE ARE USUALLY JUST AN ENCUMBRANCE
COMPLETION!
YOUR TIME WILL COME
BE SMART ABOUT IT: STAY PRIVATE
STYLE TO THE END OR YOU DON'T HAVE IT, FRIEND

CONTAGIOUS MADNESS

JUST BE NICE: CORDIAL BUT "WARM STEEL"
FALL OUT OF STRUCTURE
SEE THE SIGNS: MIXED SIGNALS OF THE SLIME
LEAVE A LEGACY THROUGH STRICT ROUTINE
COOL REJECTIONS WAKE YOU UP
CREATIVE ACT IS A STRUCTURE IN NATURE!
THE DEN OF LASCIVIOUS LIBERALISM
HAVE IMMUNITY AGAINST TYRANNY
DISCOVER WHAT YOUR KIDS ARE TAUGHT!
SIN IS NEVER SYNCHRONICITY (RIGHT SIDE OF HISTORY)
LIBERALS SAY WE'RE ALL REPLACEABLE
THE PAST IS A LESSON THAT'S ALL
MASSIVE IMMIGRATION IS DESTRUCTIVE SAVAGERY
THE CHURCHES HAVE FALLEN
"KINDNESS" IS ALWAYS THE EXCUSE
WHAT I WROTE WHEN EATING MEAT
HANDSOME AND PRETTY 1950'S
NOW: A VERY SMALL SHOPPING LIST
WOW! THIS IS HOW I'M SUPPOSED TO FEEL!
LACK OF ANIMAL FAT = INSANE (MENTALLY FLAT)
VEGAN CABAL IS LIBERAL & NEW WORLD ORDER
VEGANS LOST THEIR TEETH
POOR DECISIONS OF VEGANS
VEGAM DOCTORS: NO CREDENTIALS JUST CREDO
LOWFAT DOGMA UGLY AND DUMB?
MEAT MADE US HUMAN *AND* HUMANE
A CUTE KID BECOMES A VEGAN BIGOT
WHEN A FAT-FRUITARIAN

SEEN AS SCUM

You standing out destroys their comfort zone. It's homeostasis: maintain the system as known.

Jesus was despised and rejected by men, a man acquainted with pain and sorrows to the end.

It's stage on the Hero's Path: extreme humiliation, often public. We correct, no longer lunatic.

In some bible eras people became monsters. This is happening today: now we hear of torture.

Emotional violence broke her soul and damaged her spirit--far worse than if being beat up.

Sticks & stones break bones but words can **REALLY** hurt thee, far more consequentially.

Physical abuse is usually/often far less consequential than verbally destroying a sweet soul.

A woman is raped then cast out as despicable. The emotional assault is worse than the physical.

THE WICKED FLIP-FLOP

Wicked people are subject to changes: either from mood problems, sin or drugs/substances.

Boundaries help you sustain individual clarity. Otherwise you deflate and need them see.

Once I find out you trigger me you won't have access to me. I guard my heart and save time too see.

An insulting man comparing you to others is out of your presence, never to gain access again.

SEEN AS SCUM

Repent [stop the habit] and it breaks the past like splintered glass which then disperses at last.

They are so stupid it's hard to imagine. Distracted by sex, the taste trip or thoughts of revenge.

GOD SEES WHO YOU WILL BE

God sees who you are destined to be so protects His own even when they act indiscreetly.

God's people shall not be condemned--what does that mean? There's no memory of you as a fiend.

They can't see both sides of the gestalt at same time: past/bad vs. the present/good side.

The welfare of humanity has always been the alibi of tyrants. Albert Haye

If it's just you, without ridicule, you have it made rest of the way: success and home with view.

When young and unboundaried life escapes God. You're targeted anyway then it's a flood.

It was an upside down world where everything was my fault and bad guys were the "good".

That was way down the ladder before I knew about humans. I was an open book and lovin'.

CREEPS WORM THEIR WAY IN

They worm their way in, creeping into your house, home and head. To losers you're a magnet friend.

They are zombies with no direction: leeches, barnacles and parasites you should be rid of son.

SEEN AS SCUM

Let God vindicate you for you are His and He always takes car of/avenges His champions.

Leave hell behind. When you were used, abused: without boundaries and losing your mind.

IMPOSTOR SYNDROME

If the shame is too great we easily fall into the impostor syndrome: I don't deserve this/I'm too dumb.

They can't think nor reason, blocked by that silly imputed liberal narrative embedded in them.

One can be so traumatized the brain is blown/miswired and he's "insane", emotionally drained.

You're a kind person, concentrate on that. You're not like those creepy cowards/mean rats.

Triple Pisces is the worst or the best depending. Don't ever let the devil in or it's extreme

Boundaries mended: In the old days we slapped their faces but now we pray they won't be offended.

CHRISTIAN DIVAS?

Christian with Diva complex? If your motives are good you can be as conceited as you please.

It's like an automatic social homeostasis and yes there is a women-hating trend amongst us.

If you merely ask He rescues you from sin no matter how long you've been enslaved friend.

To the evil fray: God'll put the temptation in your way but then watch how you behave ok.

SEEN AS SCUM

Tho' swindled, God evens it out. He'll put holes in their bucket but increase your yield tenfold.

Millions are nothing to the Lord. Sometimes He takes things for a lesson but then it's all restored.

Sadly women are struggling in relationships where emotional violence is a daily occurrence.

Liberal inclusion is a blatant lie. "These are wonderful people" while rich ship em out day and night.

There is no such thing as non-binary. The whole universe bifurcates into TWO eternally.

A healthy spirit conquers adversity but what can you do when the spirit is crushed? Prov. 18

JEALOUS OF YOUR BLESSINGS

Some people just hate you cuz you're blessed: born with a silver spoon they say, pissed.

I'm not gonna stop walkin' in my blessings so you like me. If you can't handle it go climb a tree.

It's not about handling the blessing but can you handle the persecution that comes inevitably?

All your friends aren't happy when you get a new house, get engaged or are promoted at your job.

It's not so much the success but the aspiring to it since that makes man human [and God will bless}.

BREAKING DOWN THRU HUMILIATION

He meets a woman who is way up here and he breaks her down to where she's down there.

SEEN AS SCUM

A woman's spirit is broken so that they may control her. Did it happen in marriage or by your sister?

He's psychologically toying and emotionally assaulting with the constant put-downs you're hearing.

The reason for emotional violence is control, if not to show others what happens by example.

How does emotional violence break down and control you? It's humiliation it comes through.

You're not good enough, others are better, or "how's your little business doing brother?"

The emotionally violent are unpredictable. Humiliation is sporadic so you can never feel stable.

The unpredictable relationship is filled with pressure. She's losing her looks/no more a treasure.

Pressure, unpredictability, anguish: it's just words but she begins to feel she's in a grenade range.

He pushes her to do things she's not comfortable with. The overall energy of this dyad is anguish.

It's a high beauty tax when you can never relax and there's never anything but apprehensiveness.

Always waiting for the other shoe to drop knowing this will never stop. It was hell on earth God!

HUMILIATION OF DECEPTION

Deception is emotional violence. He leads her to believe a lie which then causes soul damage.

Anyone constantly deceiving is doing it intentionally. Mixed signals are part of the plan see.

SEEN AS SCUM

Constantly building up hopes but never coming thru is happening intentionally, know this Sue.

A queen's broken consciousness says "he's so deceptive I must save him"--not herself.

It is especially hurtful when it's an esteemed person who deceives you: you're sad, confused.

A dog treated like that lays down in a corner and sleeps. With confusion all energy's decreased.

A trusted spouse is found with porn or an affair. The human biocomputer breaks down, scared.

"You do it again" and he does it. "Again" and he does it again. You sink lower in your self-esteem.

OBEYING A BAD MAN IS SATAN

When deceived by a person we disobey God: that's the reason. Addicted to a sleaze you obey Satan.

The soul lays down and dies when one is constantly deceiving you with hope deferred and lies.

When things get down it's an opportunity to turn it around. Hard times = greatness found.

I felt totally misjudged in the human race and now I see the universality of it with God's Elect ok.

I had to deal with false accusation and calumny constantly from sibling rivalry in a family.

It's a giant speed bump when you can't say what you want or you can but meet an INNER block.

If you help people to think for themselves you are an enemy of the establishment and loathed.

SEEN AS SCUM

When telling the truth they try to replace you with a puppet or an oily mouthpiece stupid.

There are those with good character and those who will change overnight against you: flip floppers.

JEALOUS SUPERIORS AND FRIENDS

A higher up jealously decided you were a threat and their flying monkeys got right on it.

Those who flip flop against you cuza superior said so have no moral fiber: remember that now.

It wasn't that he was viewing pornography but that it's easy to click on the wrong thing.

Entanglement: you no longer know where this person ends and you begin, tied in knots of sin.

Boundaries preserve time. Otherwise they come in interrupting and soon the day's gone, aye.

There are silk rope vs. stonewall boundaries. Silly women allow men in their house: creepies.

Wicked men creeping into houses leading captive those women full of desires and wants/sluts.

HE KNOWS WHAT HE IS DOING

People who love you learn you. If triggering you daily it's breaching an emotional boundary.

He knows what he's sayin'. It's an intentional triggering and enslavement cuz he knows women.

A triggering man must be a hard boundary. He knows what he's saying and the reaction likely.

SEEN AS SCUM

He knows exactly what he's doing and guarding your heart is your responsibility: stop hurting.

Life starts with the heart so anyone playing with your heart [sting-shots] should have no part.

TRIGGERING YOU CONSTANTLY

Triggering you constantly, pin-pricks. He knows exactly what he's doing so exit and be perfect.

Christianity is about the individual. As such it's a giant relief felt immediately, not seeking approval.

Christians not seeking approval of the conforming collective is a threat to the establishment.

Americana is all rugged individual. Get too close and it's F-U. I like that, I'm a recluse/desert rat.

Americana is all Christian roots. It's about aspiring to the highest while with hard boundaries too.

Great works of art of the Renaissance was from individualism, not conformity or idealism.

Stiff upper lip: emotional control. Focus/boundaries: you have your goal. Pray, it's yours now.

EMOTIONAL IMMATURITY

You're not gonna fall apart again and go insane cuz you've got control of the lower brain ok?

I fell apart, crying in public and other weak and weaselly behaviors of a non-queen so unself-aware.

Christianity isn't about rigid rules and goody-goody but the individual and God above humanity.

SEEN AS SCUM

We sin as a bio-device to deal with status tension and aggression in the herd but its soul murder.

Repent of sin, get power back. Christ's atonement on cross wipes the past out: it's erased, in fact.

There is no past, it's only a dimension. What keeps it alive is sinning to avoid it in pure repetition.

Bad leaders want our allegiance to them--the whole reason they hate us: we will not bend.

THE RENAISSANCE MAN IS GONE

A free society explodes into the Renaissance Man: a genius because he's finally free again.

The drought is spiritual and mental. It's actually the same thing: dumbed by dirty disorder/devil.

Tyranny with so many restrictions [Obama/Biden's nation] blocks all creativity fast son.

The rare genius/Renaissance Man: take a look at the cathedrals, impossible in dum-dum land.

You gotta have hard boundaries around certain things. Like your kids--stop letting various men in.

It's the social hangout culture. losers without jobs creeping into weak women's houses I declare.

Don't think about that. Put a wall around those thoughts. Curb yourself, self-control, rid fat.

CALLOUSNESS OF YOUTH

They're young and it's callous and cruel. At least to me, protected & brought up in the old school.

SEEN AS SCUM

We've lost our American sensibilities invaded by foreign entities who don't love puppies & kitties.

Americans were decent law abiding people but now we hear things like beheadings in public too.

They call themselves loving but couldn't be more heedless and negligent, it's unnerving.

Most cruelty comes from negligence not from outright sadistic attacks on you or the kids.

DIS-FATTEN: SUPERFLUOUS THOUGHTS

Dis-fatten. Don't just slim down fat but also useless and repetitive thoughts: superfluous crap.

If you don't have boundaries against men it's not my fault—tell em not to come or get the hell out.

You're a guest in my home and you bring/invite your friends? Gross, low class, I'm rejectin'.

As I sit with two cats and two dogs hearing wind thru window/rain on roof I'm in heaven truly.

In high school I suffered in love, a reduplication of the early trauma, a lovesick depression.

Don't worry over past, no matter how crazy you were they always saw the genius of the situation.

And God said "that's enough writing for today, switch to music or just muse with the views ok?"

NEW AGE NERDS ESTABLISHMENT

The new establishment are new age nerds trained to think globalist with communism preferred.

SEEN AS SCUM

Due to my high energy when I went wrong it was extreme: many public mistakes without God.

I couldn't help it. Sin is possession then you see "autonomisms", uprushes of words foreign.

Americana is so individualist they'd move when one got within five miles of them in the old west.

TRIGGERING SELF-ESTEEM LEAKS

Remember this: if he's triggering your self-esteem or emotions constantly he **KNOWS** it sis.

If he's bringing you into competition with other women he **KNOWS** what he is doing: degrading.

The third world is collectivist, strict conformist and socialist/communist. My God, not us!

Just cuz they're dumb and dense you blame yourself? That doesn't seem right for a magic elf.

The inferior are always chatting together and the kings collude against God's sons/daughters.

They actually think patriotism and love of country is evil and now they're even labeling it criminal.

Stop chasing fantasies when it's just a dependency bond from early trauma you're wantin'.

Codependency is a fantasy bond never resolved. It can never give you what you want--a mirage.

Part of the syndrome is no one believes the wife of the alcoholic cuz his torture is in private.

Instead of being childlike with a myopic view [tunnel-visioned] grow up and see the broad one.

SEEN AS SCUM

Just cuz it's common doesn't mean you can forget about it after slipping and doing it so forget that.

Don't take child's view of either hate or love for one but the adult's: good and bad in perspective.

Any kind of obsession for a person is wrong and I had love addictions. Get into YOU now hon'.

Addictive devices to avoid anxiety: I was a sinner and it meant decades of human treachery.

Had a problem with women: two older sisters & mother, female logic: you know what I mean man.

Public schools are failure factory where violence is common and learning is rare/I was scared.

Weakness invites the wolves. Years ago I proved this out being invaded by a buncha evil boys.

EMOTIONAL VIOLENCE

Whether it was cuz God saves queens or for whatever reason I escaped men and learned my lesson.

In every instance when I chose to get out God gave me a hint of who to call and presto: rescued tho' still appalled.

They are mental maneuvers designed to create confusion as self-esteem spirals down.

Insecurity, self-doubt and emotional paralysis is the result of being sucked into this matrix.

Emotional violence put you in a place of indecision: being stuck, crushing the spirit like bad luck.

You may not pick it up on your spirit but the crushing effect is undeniable, feeling like hell below.

SEEN AS SCUM

America has never been united except in principals that maintain their individuality uncorrupted.

The older I get the more I have to NOT look back on while simultaneously it's all I've known.

DECEPTION IS EMOTIONAL VIOLENCE

Deception is emotional violence and that's why our self-esteem is emptied out in increments.

Deception causes us to question our intelligence. Self-denigration: calling yourself stupid or idiot.

Deception shifts how we see ourselves. An unstable environment does that to all animals.

Deception causes us to question our personal value: why would they do this to me, you know.

Deception makes us question our personal value: why do this to me? Secret coalitions from below.

A sick system with sibling abuse is defined by secret coalitions and the victim feels it all too.

Deception from past relationships prevents full trust now and that explains the endless trouble.

As a naive girl I saw deception as an annoyance but never as emotional violence which it WAS.

I saw deception as emotional violence due to the bad effects: years lost fearing what comes next.

Deception causes one to question their own intelligence. You are confused, dumbed, dense.

SILENCE IS HELLISH

SEEN AS SCUM

Silence is another device to confuse the mind. They're still stealing your space but so dam unkind.

Silence makes you second guess--you're silenced into surrender, esp. for women who are insecure.

The silent treatment is a battering ram on the heart. Talk things out, get happy again, restart.

Silence says: I'm rejecting you, you don't matter, let me show you how much you're nothing sister."

I'll be in the house but won't speak to your for days. You are rejected, on my black list ok.

Silence says: You're not worth anything, I don't know you/love you so why would I defend you.

They're silent when they know you need closure. It's mean, takes your breath away, incites fear.

Silence is like ghosting you in person. It's saying you are lower than the gum on his shoe man.

He was despised and we did not appreciate his worth or esteem him: that's how silence condemns.

SILENCE IS A RUDDER OF CONTROL

Silence is used as a rudder for control: you agree with me and we will talk, otherwise go to hell.

"What's wrong? Please tell me what's wrong." Silence says: sink in your swill/hang by your thumbs.

He knew I needed closure and answers so he purposely and sadistically closed up like an oyster.

They love it: they know you're confused and have questions and gloat in your triggered emotions.

SEEN AS SCUM

They're malicious in their satisfaction from driving you crazy and making you so dam sad man.

Watch out for MOST humans because if they are not with God they're just housing demons.

Wide is the path to hell, narrow the one to heaven: there's only a trickle who make it friend.

Silence is saying: you're invisible, you don't matter to me--a slap in the face and a message see.

Silence is like being ignored in a crowd: you're as insignificant as the paint on the walls.

She'll do ANYTHING to make him talk and not ghost her anymore. He loves that and does it more.

Are you living with one who makes you feel completely invisible? Lock your door/come alive girl.

CHAOS FROM EMOTIONAL VIOLENCE

Abused kids addicted to chaos create it constantly whether in marriage or with the boss.

By the time of nine the child is already traumatized with PTSD and a confused, warlike mind.

Adapt to chaos, brain recreates it. Adapt to a meanie and become one, knowing how to do it.

A defective biocomputer: this is what you become as you flail around searching for solutions.

Then there's angry bitterness/sadistic cleverness in driving the other into sadness and reticence.

Contrast a Vow of Silence between two married saints in the same house: a great spiritual device.

SEEN AS SCUM

Deception shifts how you see you: "I'm an idiot, I'm stupid" but self-denigration isn't cute.

Addicted to chaos: things are running fine and she throws a tantrum just like mom--she snaps.

SAVIOR ARCHETYPE BEGINS AS LOWEST ASS

Some must aspire to the highest or degrade to the lowest and become the biggest horse's asses.

The savior archetype begins as the lowest horse's ass. It's two opposites or extremes, always.

You can't help how others perceive things. No matter what they think do your own thing.

You're in a different time dimension than them. They get older but you get better to the end.

Cease seeing unique actors and see it all as archetypes. Look at forces not people [mere props].

They haven't been to war/served as cops but they have PTSD the most from emotional violence.**

CHAOS MAKERS ARE EMOTIONALLY VIOLENT

The child grows up in chaos, yelling, hate and fighting. Addicted to chaos it even evokes laughing.

Addicted to chaos they transport it into your life. Shut them out now or stay with the devil/strife.

With this person you have anxiety and high blood pressure. You're sleeping less/eating more.

Now you need a therapist with this chaotic creep. It's better to be alone and happy/don't you see.

SEEN AS SCUM

Make no friendship with an angry man, with a furious man do not go. Keep this characters out now.

Keep him out lest you learn his ways: a snare to your SOUL—you mind, will and emotions.

Wringing my hands, wondering what I did, stunned at the suddenness, feeling inferior, self-disgust.

He's not going to apologize when older cuz he's gotten more evil when older: don't expect closure.

CHAOS CREATES SOUL TIES

Chaos creates soul ties. Life in dysfunction is addiction to adrenalin from deferred hope and lies.

Living with her diva complex means you stay down in the impostor syndrome in a perfect fit.

Constantly creating issues and situations that don't matter: exit the hell from this chaos-maker.

Recognize chaos as emotional violence. Think of your nervousness/fears in solar plexus/guts.

Reject anyone who disrupts your peace. See demonic effects of even having em around, please.

Friends? Mad with the world, blowing their horn, road rage, arguing with the waitress, revenge.

INVALIDATION IS VIOLENCE

Invalidation is also emotional violence. This person trivializes your feelings, intellect, existence.

They have no empathy when you're hurting and will NOT recognize your accomplishments surely.

SEEN AS SCUM

"Just get over it--grow up". Invalidating your feelings is emotional violence but it's cultural/dense.

Emotional invalidation is painful. Whether intentional or not it is abuse and creates havoc tomorrow.

It's an art form of some to minimize people. If you don't like it and he does it again it's intentional.

You're excited about a new project, they put a lid on it. It's a letdown and abuse so remove the twits.

Rejoice with those who rejoice. If they don't get excited for you they must lose access to you sis.

At critical points they shame you or bring up the past. It's a losing game with emotional violence.

BLAME-SHIFTING IS VIOLENCE

Blame Shifting: they accuse you for failures. It's all your fault and they camp in your guilt forever.

Grown children who are still blaming you for the divorce and other grudges from decades before.

Chaos-addicts find stable husbands boring. This is so common today, it's bad boys they're adoring.

If you have a bad dad then transfer to a good lad and start a new wonderful life so glad.

If you had an evil sister transfer to a Christian friend cuz Jesus said they're true family to the end.

Turning your back on bad people is a most spiritual thing to do and now your light shines too.

You become the sacrifice as they blame you for everything, a scapegoat for earthlings.

SEEN AS SCUM

If you don't catch yourself you believe you are the cause of everything they come up with.

VIOLENCE OF DISACKNOWLEDGEMENT

They won't own the things they did to hurt you. They won't apologize and thus: you stay blue.

They just move on like it's all ok. They spit in your face one day then show up all smiling & friendly.

It's emotionally violent and abusive if they won't own this: a mixed signal and contradiction sis.

You're afraid to be alone so tolerate this stuff, grinning and bearing it. You give in to the twits.

Acknowledgement: You're not gonna hurt me in a significant way & not even talk about it.

It's impossible to be settled with a person who covers his transgressions: we can't go on man.

Even if you love em to stay with em you must devalue yourself. He cheats, you stay, you pay.

Constantly threatening to leave unless you obey--that's emotional violence and manipulation ok.

Who are you threatening to leave me anyway? Here's money/get the hell outa here buddy.

OLDER IS OUTA TURMOIL AND TORTURE

Younger means embroiled in the turmoil described above, older is having these things resolved.

Don't ever look at it thru their eyes, only your own. This relieves guilt and shame imputed without.

SEEN AS SCUM

Everyone has their boring little thing, they don't care about your universal/historical discoveries.

Some people are good, some are bad, some are bad for awhile and then come back: don't split.

It is the bio-instincts [food/sex] that become compulsive as energy is recycled in outworn channels.

Instead of the energy rising up to the head conquering the situation it floods into lower affections.

PLAYING VICTIM IS THE MODERN CURSE

Playing victim is the modern curse. Other than that it's all about her and these aren't queenly sir.

Legends good/bad die hard in families. Sometimes you just gotta relocate to be yourself today.

Re-elevate, adjust your mood today: see experience as self-achieved and enjoy every minute ok.

Your work stands on it's own--you don't have to go out there and defend it unless its poorly done.

Misjudged constantly, seeing inferiors placed ahead of me: I got used to it and I'm a whitey.

Having suffered boundary and moral collapse I know what it's like in fact: your world goes black.

MISJUDGEMENT BY INFERIORS

I got used to constant misjudgment by inferiors in control and it was depressing ya' know.

I got the opportunity to see what it's like. Being hated by one then the whole group joins in, aye.

SEEN AS SCUM

You get used to misjudgment and it's a guarded, lower state. I'd smoke pot in my room to elevate.

In that era I felt severely misjudged every minute--had to achieve a better carriage to be above it.

They explain in long treatises what the silly painting meant. It should stand on its own friend.

It was like getting hit men to do her dirty work. Just gossiping to the wrong person is dangerous.

LIBERALS THINK ALL ARE GOOD

Liberals think we're all good/anything bad is justified by childhood: empty prisons/love the hoods.

How life works: if friends you disconnect they may not be there when you come back in fact.

She's your greatest booster, inadvertently. You excelled to dispel her public shaming constantly.

You get on a tangent and suddenly the whole day's gone. Brain tracked, self-esteem down.

Superior thoughts are in you already so why distract from those with inferior past times/studies?

Turn it all off and stop filling your head with lesser things than what God put in there instead.

God, because You are One who puts down my enemies it is You I will worship today/always.

They don't want an apology, they want public humiliation. Calumny, opprobrium.

CLOWNS ARE RUNNING THE CIRCUS

SEEN AS SCUM

The clowns are running the circus. Now they're saying men get pregnant and they're serious.

They're like anybody's family: prodigal sons, miscreants, wrong mate selectors, treachery.

She's a fake humanitarian/feminist, a social climber abusing her celebrity in the royal family.

The very idea that you can solve race obsession with more race obsession is a terrible notion.

"BE LIKE US, THE GOOD PEOPLE"

"Be like us because we are good people". That's all we heard from the young royals, so dull.

They're sure they're right cuz it's what they heard and everyone else thinks it too: that's the herd.

Talking loud and arrogant, standing out or interrupting, using superior sarcasm: that's them man.

You're so dam arrogant, shut the fruit up. That's what we all think when we hear those broads.

The female narcissist can't see her Diva Complex. It's even attractive to some despite bad effects.

When an arrogant female embarrasses you cuz she's so out of order that's the Diva Disorder.

The self-imploding Diva Complex in politician women is because they haven't studied the men.

WOMEN SHOULD STUDY MEN

Women should study men: how they think and act. Not impose themselves with a Diva Complex.

SEEN AS SCUM

Virtue's cost is high above rubies--it's gonna cost him something--so then it's appreciated see.

Virtue never chases and it does not catch. Virtue is pursued, virtue approves and is caught too.

Virtue in the eyes of the man is "wife swag". The slut is a virtual nobody and potentially a nag.

The only way she can attach is to sacrifice her body but a man is attached to virtue not immorality.

Every man is attracted sexually on some level but to attract a man is not attaching one.

MEN BOND IN PURSUIT

He pulls away cuz men bond in pursuit. When not given that opportunity he wants space not you.

He's pretty good at what he does, she calls it love and a soul tie develops: kept low with him above.

The chasing female is broken from previous traumas so the bait she uses bites her in the butt.

He wants space until invested, which happens in the pursuit but that's not happening too.

She wants to get closer but he wants his space. Post-orgasmic withdrawal is next always.

Here's the problem: when a woman has sex she wants to bond [get closer] just as he dumps her.

Fact: A woman who chases is reduced to using sex cuz to chase but not catch looks foolish.

She has to disregard her morals, disrespect her virtue and dishonor her body to catch at all.

SEEN AS SCUM

Out of natural order, you chase/catch but how to maintain a mismatch? Think on this lass.

He pursues, she approves. You can get him temporarily hooked through sex but it won't continue.

Chase and catch: a chasing woman must potentially disregard her morals in order to catch.

A man is not impressed [enough to get on the hook] by anything other than sex so that's the gist.

CHASERS NEVER SEEN AS PRIZE

Chasers are treated as game and never honored as the prize. You're just a fish in the net, aye.

To "catch" a man is to grasp and control him and what is her bait? It's been sex from the beginning.

He pursues, she approves. He pursues more, she approves more until connection is true.

The whole ecosystem of the relational process is thrown into a whirlwind when she chases ok.

A woman who chases is convinced her value is too low to expect to be pursued: its an undertow.

Chasing pacifies in the moment without the existential experience of being desired and sought.

To chase is to misrepresent/dishonor herself. Hearing the clock ticking she welcomes hell.

MASSIVE GENDER CONFUSION

Massive identity confusion: men behaving like women and visa versa--of course she chases ya.

SEEN AS SCUM

Refusing to know God they soon didn't know how to be human [man or woman] either. Romans 1: 26

The mere decision collects data needed to escape. You'll be surprised at God's clever ways.

Heal thyself: plan to get out. Just that alone sets the brain in a new direction powered by God.

With a decreasing sense of value, she chases. That stunts her more in embarrassing phases.

Broken consciousness is a sense of decreasing value. For a woman it's the end and it's terrible.

FREEDOM TO SIN IS SLAVERY

Freedom [to sin] is not freedom but slavery: tho' it seems like independence one isn't happy.

They criminalize dissent, weaponize the legal and redefine half of us as national security threat.

Pisces feel things on deep spiritual levels so triple Pisces, get busy and reject the devil.

Some are damaged forever as memory locks in the cells and muscles like the event is here/now.

Life is a ladder and I came from way down there. Don't think back because it acts like an anchor.

Healthy background: Safety, tools/resources, parents healed from trauma, discipline but love.

Materialism, social media & reality TV were triple threats turning everyone into narcissists.

FALSE ACCUSATIONS AND COLDNESS

SEEN AS SCUM

She who is most sensitive to contradiction will go most crazy with mixed signals/cold situations.

The stress of living under false accusation was too much to take hon'. Have a good life: so long.

Left wing activists disguised as journalists make the same old tired accusation of patriots.

You will no longer infect our children with your woke rot. It's over, admit it and resign or just bow out.

They call you ungrateful: because you hate being shafted & gouged the independent are called out.

MATURITY: GHOST ME AND GOODBYE

A sign of maturity: ghost me and I'll simply remove you from my address book--have a good day.

Luckily life is in phases so now you're done with a rudderless life of reactive not creativeness.

Luckily life is in phases so now you're done with siblings who are envious, jealous and hateful.

Replace shame with fame, for it is the same bold audacity creating both waves so do it ok?

It's not that you have so many enemies but the hedge is down so you're a dam pin cushion see.

You've a vision of cornucopia but start to drink again then their reactions complete your descent.

WOMEN HATING WOMEN TREND

The women were mean too/the worst. Sting-shots and flip-flops, I was an unprotected target.

SEEN AS SCUM

I'm hypersensitive to mice or men and losing my hedge of protection was hell on earth man.

When I lost the penthouse I was surrounded by the anti-woman mob, a pin-cushion/it was sudden.

You gotta teach a constant vetting system. Good or evil, learn to see the differences ma'am.

Assuming everyone is "good". What a danger to teach when evil predominates even in childhood.

It was like putting a rattlesnake in my cage. You never know if we can mix, it's a sign of new age.

What I know now: I'm super-sensitive to people and ridicule and desperately need solitude.

The trauma of betrayal collapses morals and we do stupid and despicable things that's all.

NEED CONVALESCENCE AFTER MESS

You need time to heal from rejection, abandonment, trauma. It's a rough ride on the lower rung.

I'm trying to save precious lives from the most vile people. When I was young I saw no evil.

My ancestors were either great orators drawing crowds or drunk in the gutter and nothing other.

Don't EVER explain yourself to them. The bible speaks of child-bearing women but also the barren.

I love the feeling every moment is mine without having to adapt to anyone-- that's called hateful hon'.

Now safely relocated and behind a locked gate I'm in heaven every minute: no surprises ok.

SEEN AS SCUM

Without a fence I had to put up with their invasions, always saying "hey, someone is coming."

THE SOCIAL IMPOSE THE LOW

This generation is SOCIAL and that means they bring their friends and triangulate/you go low.

If the only way to get their claws outa ya/stop talking is to relocate that alone proves this theory.

California cops were coddling teens in the eighties: not arresting for broken windows/trespassing.

When a hammer everything's a nail and Biden just hired 87,000 tax agents to make sure you fail.

Get ready: your hero's about to deflate--will his depedestalization crush your trusting spirit?

The philistines can't see how gross, vulgar and imposing they are so adapting to them is a terror.

Invading my home with your army/entourage was the height of your rudeness jezebel witch.

You bringing strangers here was the height of your rudeness: being your friend was high stress.

Bait and switch is bullsh*t. You give an estimate and that's what I pay, not add on later you twit.

House with fence: you can't get to me anymore like when I was in an apt. on the ground floor.

CRISIS CREATES BATTLESHIP

After 31 years a new comportment style was encrypted into my DNA--at least it feels that way.

SEEN AS SCUM

It was the combo of people imposing on me constantly with the heat making it hard to eat/sleep.

If I hadn't gone thru all that I'd be an ordinary entitled brat, a weak/loosely organized battleship.

The explosion of surplus potentials in problem areas: that's why we don't have resentments.

GENIUS BRED IN PROBLEM ENVIRONMENTS

Genius is bred in problem environments triggering those characteristics: adapt or be a lunatic.

The extreme heat coupled with no fence or gate served to aggravate then make me a certain way.

God put me in extreme conditions like 120 degree heat to tighten/toughen my style and routines.

Her vindictiveness knew no bounds. She didn't keep it in the family either/spread it all around.

Relocate: I've a right to be proud of who I am today, free of yesterday and all what they say.

Anything that isn't you is gonna crash and burn. The fake identity implodes/has a bad outcome.

WITCHES/ADULTERERS HANG TOGETHER

The adulterers, witches and slanderers hang together. They gossip about you, birds of a feather.

Sex is the path of least resistance cuz it's easiest. Restraint and decency requires strength sis.

A woman who does not make God her Rock is immoral: she goes along with the flock.

SEEN AS SCUM

New doors open when we [eliminate]: leave a space. It's pneumaticity: it all fills in new today.

TRAUMA AND LOST BOUNDARIES

Trauma: lost both parents in her thirties then husband became alcoholic, her worst enemy.

Explanation of bad times of life: the hedge was down and evil's the default setting all around.

God doesn't want you scared like this. He doesn't want you thinking of the morbid past much either sis.

Despite smear campaigns you still win: as the foes die, move away/forget but you're now perfect.

You get use to getting no attention so the first one who does sweeps you off your feet tho' a skuzz.

It's the Dunning-Kruger Effect of the dumb thinking they're smart. Dealing with this is an art.

This comes from trauma: thinking you can change him. If only you're nice enough or a good friend.

Are you still masochistically attracted to men who are only into themselves, never reaching out?

HOW INSANE YOU GOT ADAPTING TO ROT

I don't care how insane you got adapting to rot it's water under the bridge: you were just a tot.

The biggest mal-adaptation of the wife of the alcoholic is to get drunk herself, blamed to hell.

If they don't understand you anyway and then they hear shit they fill their cup with it. KK on twits

SEEN AS SCUM

Don't blame them for hell you went thru due to sin: an inevitable process which is not about them.

MAL-ADAPTATION TO ENVIRONMENT

We mal-adapt to our environment and that becomes the mental illness we have to heal from.

The family as system splits between the scapegoat and the narcissist with flying monkey backup.

Inherited shame [I.S.] is like a boulder coming down the bloodline pike to land on ONE poor tyke.

Inherited shame is like wearing slime. You wake up each morning wondering why you're even alive.

Centuries of a bloodline's shame shit pile falls onto ONE. Inherited shame is a terrible thing son.

The hurt & trauma went so deep it pierced the mystic center and out came divine nectar: words.

Silence is a cure for grief. It always bring us back to self/God as we start on a path of relief.

To be misjudged can cause mental illness as frustration leads to aggression then control by twits.

After caving in you gotta get strong again. This time no matter what you don't mal-adapt thru sin.

DECEPTIVE BETRAYALS MAKE US CRAZY

He made you crazy with his deceptive betrayals then blamed you for everything after all.

In smear campaigns speculation overwhelm evidence and it's blown up to pure hellishness.

SEEN AS SCUM

You know why we're a king and queen? Cuz we've relocated and behind a locked gate see.

Rising up triggers inherited shame from others and the result is blocked success/relapse to gutter.

As we rise up inherited shame [I.S.] kicks in. This is the stuff imputed from jealous others again.

I caved in, like I was muted for years. They aren't just speed bumps they screw your mind up.

A SLUT OR JUST BOUNDARILESS?

Was she a slut or just boundaryless? Cuz molestation is the default setting without em I insist.

I was attacked for not saying he "and she" but "he" is a nonpersonal pronoun re: ALL mankind.

Being younger was a great danger. No boundaries, a naive truster targeted by haters/womanizers.

They are traumatized lemmings. That's why they cling, grab and get violent if you ask for privacy.

If he's your husband/she's your wife you will connect cuz it's God's will and good for the Elect.

Their notion of compassion has nothing to do with you. You can stew cuz their ideas you refuse.

Don't fret calumnious attacks--killing your rep--cuz if not true they lose all foundation, so relax.

n fear of her vicious tongue or gossiping even more, I didn't confront the Jezebel destroyer.

In fear of survival I flattered the opinion leader or gossiper to put an end to the matter.

SEEN AS SCUM

Without judge or jury: they take all allegations about you very seriously but about them, never.

As due process breaks down people will believe what they hear without judge nor jurors.

The good book says women aren't to rule the church/not to chatter in the sanctuary either.

CRAZY OR FERTILE ANARCHY?

They called me crazy but it was just fertile anarchy. An inside job and my Ph.D. in the streets see.

Old church was always on guard against heresy but with leaven-creep it isn't the way it is today.

If there's an undertow get healthy/stay high by simply staying away. That's your therapy.

How to be a modern yogi with longevity: simply stay away. Eccentric loners live longer they say.

You burned your house down or divorced the wrong man: the hero's path but you're back again.

Even if they got you drunk, raped you then blamed you for it--it was part of the hero's path sis.

My dry years were a fertile anarchy inside, often manifested in confusion or being schizoid.

STAGE OF BLOSSOMING

But after years of tribulation the flower finally blossoms and all things come together: oh man!

Churches are full of new age leaven and much of it's due to the paganism of ruling women.

SEEN AS SCUM

Much of the creative act is fertile anarchy: feels like confusion inside but still creative see.

Born clear we come into a system that awaits us. We adapt thru blindness until self-awareness.

Just cuz you had dry years doesn't mean you weren't doing anything. It's an inside evolution see.

Sin puts you under the control of peons, thru shame. It's the devils game and humiliating.

YOU HAD TO EXPERIENCE BEDLAM

You're WAY up now cuz you were WAY down then: life is a ladder/you had to experience bedlam.

The cops hauling you off, being the black sheep talk of the town, being smeared like a clown.

Stop remorsing. Spending a night in jail may be part of the hero's path or being down for months

Stop bemoaning the past when you didn't know what was going on/led by instinct and crowds.

I finally saw it didn't matter what they think, just dumb twits and moths in the night see.

The thought of having to adapt to those people is too horrible to imagine and I did it man.

Deep state has unleashed forces in maga party that will not stop until the dems lie in ruins, sorry!

Men and kids don't leave home so much if the wife/mom makes it interesting, orderly, clean, fun.

These are not the days of JFK, "democrat/liberal" don't mean what they use to mean ok.

SEEN AS SCUM

Skeletons yelling at us, those in the closet, gossiped about by those closest: all people pests.

Ruminating listening to music/looking out the window is the most fruitful past time you know

Being treated like crap on the way up is part of the Hero's Path. Don't resent, it's a process.

BORN CLEAR, WE MAL-ADAPT

Born clear, we mal-adapt to the system which awaits us. Often it's just too awful to imagine it.

The past broke down like an evil fairytale with cartoon actors teaching me all I needed to know.

Inherited shame is a trip laid on you. You can accept or reject it but you're usually too young to.

When it's all social--who's superior to who--there's no right-brained enjoyment of the moment.

Inherited shame it's called: They laid a trip on us and it formed a low ceiling of success for us all.

These skeletons are shaming us and we're taking it on with self-disgust. Think deeply on this.

At the basis of psychology is skeletons. In our past, yelling at us, influencing good/bad actions.

MANAGING COMMIE SIBLING ATTACKS

I didn't know how to handle it. They came back from liberal universities all accusatory/twits.

After being so nice at first she suddenly started attacking me and it was hell on earth see.

SEEN AS SCUM

Smear campaigns produce intended results. Without judge nor jury all believe family pundits.

I'm always praying today it all bursts open. It's a fifty year project with one paycheck in the end.

How do skeletons relate to psychology? A lot: ancestry coming out and skeletons in the closet.

Liberals: As long as it's not happening to them and palliated by CNN they don't care about you man.

ARCHETYPES ARE STUFF OF FAIRYTALES

Tho' archetypes are the stuff of fairytales it's how we see the world: through caricatures.

We don't "see" a person, the brain puts him in a category. Archetypes are these caricatures see.

What a nightmare it was to be the target of her projection. It's the jungle mentality son.

How interesting: God punishes enemies on basis of what you're destined in the future to be.

The stress level is too high if you can't forgive as you also hang onto memories and get sick.

Once dropping outa family lockstep it's hard as you aren't really connected so go no contact.

In prayer, ask then get off of it. Don't waste God's time, no chanting: He'll get right on it.

CORNUCOPIA LIGHTS UP WHEN...

The cornucopia lit up ONLY when doing my own thing while locking the gate and not caring ok.

SEEN AS SCUM

I had to learn what boundarilessness was like. Those were dry years of sad darkness in the night.

Weakness invites aggression. You were a fool to let em in so they took it out on you: it's a system.

Modern sex ed is nothing but cartoon porn. Must face it: pornography for kids is the new norm.

San Diego teachers can no longer say "men/women" but "people with a penis/vulva", no kidding.

San Diego Schools claim heterosexuality is a system of oppression so genders must be examined.

Queer theory states that the gender binary is just a social construct and thus harmful to society.

The real you steps forward as impostor disperses. It's based on hard work for years and you did it.

Let creativity & tenacity give you status, not climbing with approval-getting, a waste of time.

When you empower the least talented among us giving them unchecked power they take over.

There's an UNDERTOW we gotta mitigate against. To not know that is immaturity/boundarilessness.

ON THE FOOD NOTE, NEW THOUGHTS

Smoothies between meals is not intermittent fasting. Just the ONE meal then water or nothing.

The one daily meal for intermittent fasting is usually a four-hour window not a one-shot deal.

Red Salad is fruit: tomatoes, red bells, zucchini sliced on romaine with olive oil/lemon too.

SEEN AS SCUM

I believe that exercise makes you look better naked but then so does alcohol. John Kennedy

I take him his tacos at noon but other than that leave him alone after ordering his office/room.

A million die in sleep from choking each year. Since it isn't always discerned it's surely far more.

Would you want two big tumors hanging off your chest? It's udderly ugly the big implant requests.

SRIs: Anti-depressants aren't happy pills but entry into a dark world and anti-psychotics even kill.

Aliesthenic hunger turn off: When the micronutrients [not calories] reach a level the hunger's gone.

Stuffed Belgian Waffle maker [WAFFLEIZER] can be used with anything like cheese/tomato/zucchini.

If food makes you choke why ever eat it? It's the new 3rd category of ED: just smoothies/juice it.

INVASION OF MILLIONS

Biden never makes the same mistake twice. He makes it five or six times just to be sure, aye.

They say "join Biden" in open borders, abortions up to birth, inflation, killing energy independence.

Make us poor, bring IN the poor to then install the democrats as the permanent ruling class.

We're becoming like the 3rd world: no rule of law, all is politicized and opponents are criminalized.

Give backup facts and they put a wall up while nodding as if they're in agreement: the lemmings.*

SEEN AS SCUM

"You're not a lesbian but a woman trapped in a man's body. It's not your fault, just need surgery."

VP Harris says "no border crisis" while millions come across illegally but what are we to say.

The pollution is trivial from meat compared to jet setting around the world promoting bug cuisine.

It's celebrity culture dressing itself up in global liberal causes always virtue signaling to the masses.

If you wanna make a giant even larger, raid his house: thanks to the FBI it'll now all turn around.

FAILED FAR LEFT POLICIES

American's can't afford another year of failed far left policies. With high cost energy they'll freeze.

Border states deal with millions of immigrants see while sanctuary cities buckle with fifty.

Shipping immigrants to us rich is a "holocaust" but clogging poor border towns is ok with us.

It's not a stunt. They incentivized illegal immigration so they should have to live with the situation.

They want a permanent underclass and voting block so they invite the third world to lock it up.

The signs of the times are dire. The buildup is very concerning to those of us who are clear.

If you double the price of something then lower it ten percent please don't celebrate that.

External conflicts breed internal solidarity: a most important concept in political psychology.

SEEN AS SCUM

Communism never dies, it's gets rebranded. Climate change, green new deal or inflation banned.

TRUMP DERANGEMENT SYNDROME IN WOMEN

Because I love Trump she hates me all of a sudden in a giant flip-flop but I'm ok, it's a good test run.

The purveyors of misinformation make millions while the truthseekers are banished/made irrelevant.

She has TDS so bad. She wants to kill Trump and kill me just because I like him, that's a fact.

Destruction, war, collapse, starvation, extinction: the loving liberals just love these things.

We're so unproductive with high regulations flooding the market with Biden. Sleepy get alongs.

Like all countries all through history we had slavery but unlike them all we beat it back see.

They seek to degrade our life of decency and harmony into a grim angry world of vile complaining.

We're supposed to purge our traditions & values to keep the loudest voices happy: self-treachery.

CANCEL CULTURE CATASTROPHE

Cancel culture, the military wing of wokism, is strangling American culture of the meaning of her.

You are not free if you cannot say what you think. As a human you must express yourself see.

They feel superior and don't care what we think. Can't fix stupid but we can vote it out see.

SEEN AS SCUM

The water won't clear up 'til we get the pigs outa the creek. Must throw the bums out speedily.

I believe love is the answer, I really do. But you ought to own a handgun just in case too.

BIDEN BLUES

It was a speech of a dictator--in style, visuals, words--in Biden's Enemies of the State speech.

They said it: their main enemy are republicans, veterans, gun owners, election questioners.

This is so incredibly dangerous and white conservative Christians are the target of this set up.

You could take a Jew's cow, you could disrobe his wife in public and chase her all around.

Once a group is maligned by the leader you can do anything you want to them, it's ok sir.

Those who've sold out to evil are weak. Coming from weak families they're sad/desperate see.

Their clear move is saying we're the violent ones. They always accuse us of what they're doin'.

Every country on earth had slavery thru history but it's only Americans who are blamed see.

Only America went to war to free slaves but WE are blamed by the smug liberals so accusatory.

They worship the sun god, the wind god, the god of wishful thinking & utopian envisioning.

LIBERALS CODDLE CRIMINALS NOT VICTIMS

SEEN AS SCUM

In California teens could break your windows and vandalize your home without repercussions.

Once young thugs saw the cops wouldn't protect me they took over completely, their heyday.

Young thugs leave cities to take over small towns and due to the ACLU, with no repercussions.

It's no longer about fighting crime but siding with the criminal, giving em support from us all.

In Borrego Springs they took the side of petty vandals and thieves rather than the victims see.

Signs of society screwed: Men get weak, leaders decadent, cops politicized, currency devalued.

NAZI GERMANY SHOWS PSYCHOLOGY

A group takes power, goes after foes with legal force then criminalizes all opposition of course.

Germans didn't know about the camps but they sure as hell turned against Jewish neighbors, alas.

The kids were stunned to discover those throwing rocks at their windows were beloved neighbors.

Hate always comes from below so would you change places with these foes? Always: hell no.

Hitler was not a nationalist--they don't kill their own people. He was a psychopath and sadist.

So many women are alike: hating Trump but they don't know why. Ask em questions, no reply.

Vilification of his opponents is triggering violence but that's exactly how liberals/Biden does it.

SEEN AS SCUM

Intellectual honesty and consistency is not something the left cares about: it's frustrating for us.

Since Biden, illegal got-aways number 4 million so how is the border closed like they're sayin'?

A plumber has to pay for your education to make more money: is this fair? Liberal baloney.

AFFLUENT LIBERALS WIN BIG

Their jokes stink but when the audience objects they just blame Trump supporters see.

Dare defend yourself against false accusation and get fired for creating a hostile work environment.

They criminalize dissent--weaponizing the legal--and redefine half of us as a national security threat.

We're conditioned to see racism as coming from whites just as antiwhiteism hits new heights.

Woke comedians turned political hacks have a weird power over young minds ignoring facts.

Democrat's pro-criminal policies have made warzone cities and still liberals are blind to fallacy.

Don't look at our cities, they're in shambles. Trash, crime, disorder, plight of the homeless.

RECAP OF SEEN AS SCUM

From a forest into a tree. Too many details, too much complexity: put it all in a folder and retire see.

I felt the earth shake when God was mad and don't ever wanna experience that again, so sad.

SEEN AS SCUM

I want freedom from details: retirement. I wanna divorce this huge project of a life, amen.

Instead of arguing with strangers over stupid crap seek great minds with whom to connect.

Don't think about/conger up the past cuz it's an anchor back down the ladder and what a mess!

God's favor on your life will stir up jealousy and it's dangerous cuz they'll do anything see.

THE TEST IS HANDLING PERSECUTION

You can't have the blessing without persecution cuz envy/jealousy are biggest human emotions.

If you can handle the persecution then God trusts you with the blessing: gotta pass the testing.

Pass the test of overlooking insults--they wouldn't be talking if you weren't making a difference.

Let God take care of those trying to make you look bad. They literally can't handle your success lad.

You have to be ok with them not being ok with you. Your time is too valuable/get a new crew.

You don't need all to celebrate you. Give up these notions and do your work in devotion too.

If you look to people you'll spend all your time getting their approval so that needs removal.

Never impose yourself, they should be pulled. It's a natural gravitation to the truth in you.

FIFTY YEAR PROJECT IS DONE

SEEN AS SCUM

I'm DONE. Decades-long Creative Act is complete: I'm on the beam, ocean going thru my veins it seems.

What got er done? How did you create a masterpiece? It's all by daily diligence and a vision see.

Trauma for decades: I digested it all, made a theory of it and turned it all back/makes me the Ace.

I'm the queen cuz no one can get to me. If I'm out there unprotected by walls I have no liberty.

Bliss is: freedom from interference. Because left to ourselves we are the best there is.

Taking time off is never a loss, as you go into the right brain of timeless adventure and success.

We all have a unique genius, perhaps an art form never seen before--so just work, wait and persevere.

Instead of feasting on your success day try fasting with it: as a cornucopia alights it's higher ok.

All I know after all these years is good is rewarded and bad is punished by our Father the Lord.

USE CHRISTIAN RESTRAIN THEN PAINT

Stay close to God with Christian restraint cuz things can change suddenly and you're up a creek.

Years of false accusation/being looked down upon: things have reversed, I'm on top now.

Withdraw from evil and do good. Seek peace and pursue it. Commit plans to Him, you've won.

When it comes to swindlers no one's worst than the virtue signalers/the continuous one-uppers.

SEEN AS SCUM

Period of experimentation: the hero's path is trying on friends and family but it ends eventually.

You're going uphill: closer to heaven/upward in your profession. It's not a battle, just takes skill.

All who came against you are gone or dead. It's a brand new era with you at the helm instead.

RETIREMENT IS RETURN TO CHILD

Retirement is like being a child again: psychosis, cosmic consciousness and infantilization.

I've done my best and I've gone over it again, again and once more. I'm done, so light I could soar.

With completion I still put things into place and eliminate what doesn't belong: all upward now.

Having given birth I await the LINK to success. It's how it works according to Koestler on genius.

The Creative Act has been birthed, I've returned to a child like at first--from this work I've divorced.

Relocate, get to a safe place. Dig in, gear up: the time has come to face facts tho' it hurts ok.

Let God vindicate you/even things up. He's your Champion so forgive them and He must.

The elder's last journey is a vision quest cuz he doesn't have that many wonderful minutes left.

The superior genotype of humans is genius and the reward for persecution is privacy at last.

Better impostor syndrome than diva complex don't you think? Just learn to act/maintain humility.

SEEN AS SCUM

All day and night long the superior man puts things into place or clarifies the matrix: he eliminates.

In old age we mine the past for gems. Eldering is having time for that and the self-awareness it brings.

The purpose of science is to challenge orthodoxy and dogma but that's exactly what is banned see.

Weakness of attitude is weakness of character. Albert Einstein

CONTAGIOUS MADNESS

Diet and Herd Obstructions

They didn't treat you like you were special, unique, with talent or that your emotions were significant.

You're treated with indifference/love is conditional. They compare you to others like you're fullabull.

They didn't treat you like you were special, unique, with talent or that your emotions were significant.

You're treated with indifference/love is conditional. They compare you to others like you're fullabull.

TRAUMA AND BOUNDARIES

Due to trauma you let a snake in. You wanted company/to feel alive again but he did you in.

Dear Lord please help me to recover from these memories of when trauma broke boundaries.

When the evil world flowed in and I couldn't defend myself having been muted by relatives.

In that era it seemed no one took my side and the whole world assumed I was the bad guy, aye.

It's all the result of lost hedge of protection, the process of regression into destruction from sin.

CONTAGIOUS MADNESS

I lived in fear of people calling my relatives whose only goal was to throw me to the wolves.

NASTY PROJECTIONS

Outa their dirty, filthy, nasty minds liberals accuse sweet-saint you of most debauched crimes.

Once you're pegged they fill their cup with it. Tho' you're the most clever you wear that tag forever.

The greatest example/epitome of this identity screwjob was what they did to President Trump.

Then they all jump on the bandwagon. Tho' they don't know how to think they're lemmings man.

There were years of being misjudged, mislabeled and muted--unable to stand against the foolish.

It's a false/unfair comparison to say I felt like a Jew in Nazi Germany but that was the feeling see.

Once mis-pegged in the family by vindictive jealous sisters it spread out in concentric circles.

Listen you: you don't know what I went thru or what your father went thru so shut up fool.

SELF-SERVING FAMILY MYTHS

All family myths center on them and their great achievements/worthless accomplishments.

All family patterns shut her out. The price of being different/refusing to conform has fallout.

She falls into an emotional drought, an inner vacuity that hurts like hell, an empty shell, ouch.

CONTAGIOUS MADNESS

Her mal-adaptation may be a badness role, even a slut--a common reaction seeking to be consoled.

She was relieved to know it was a mental illness not badness. Not vanity but complete madness.

Like a shunned wolf who dies of starvation, it hurts to be ostracized from the pack son.

You gotta be strong and close to your Father to deal with that, being shunned from the pack.

Once you see how cruel people can be--and not just "bad seeds"--you will grow up suddenly.

NEGLECT CREATES MENTAL ILLNESS

Neglect creates mental illness in middle agers. Tho' bad in childhood its addictions and suicide later.

In ageist societies people are neglected just cuz they aged. Youthism is destructive that way.

Before I found God as companion I could feel brain cells diminishing due to the neglect I was experiencing.

Get a robot vacuum or you're sick from pet dander and dust mites tho' you only know it later.

BRAIN-SHRINK FROM SHUN-STINK

Before God was my constant companion I felt brain cells diminishing from your neglect son.

Before God was my only family I felt my brain shrinking from ageist neglect by the untrustworthy.

If not dependent on God your life will end lopsided and up and down in wild vacillations son.

CONTAGIOUS MADNESS

If dependent on people for approval identity's on quicksand as fame turns to shame: this is crucial.

Before going no-contact I felt brain shrinking every time I thought of them: neglect/contradiction.

With early neglect the child has no identity, sense of protection or comfort. It's just a gut ache Lord.

If the adult person had loving beginnings it makes middle age neglect that much more excruciating.

AGEIST NEGLECT STARTS EARLY

Middle/old age neglect: who cares about it? No one as the lonely sinks in his swill/puts up with it.

We're losing brain cells due to painful neglect--that's a helluva concept when you think about it.

Learn to love being alone til your prefer that. It's an inner journey of adventure & enlightenment.

Once you're hep to the superiority of solitude it'll made you mad when frenemies inevitably intrude.

I am losing brain cells and it's serious. I can't remember a thing but maybe its cosmic consciousness?

And God said: "Let me show you what it feels like to have God's hand [on my shoulder] removed"

When God's hand was removed I was literally thrown to the wolves as evil flowed in like a wave.

He/she couldn't stop doing the things that made him/her ugly. That one sin came first see.

FORGIVE OR HATE YOURSELF

CONTAGIOUS MADNESS

I couldn't forgive myself until I forgave others then I was finally released from intrusive memories.

If I bring up a bad resentment to chew on I also recall the immature things I did so long ago.

What is forgiveness but finally living in the present? Not being held down by memories, little anchors.

If I forgave others, as hard as it was, I could forgive myself for flaws and embarrassing faux pas.

When he says something as self-serving/sensual as that don't think you're gonna change a dirty rat.

To be hurt cuz he wants privacy is immature, emotional, feminine cuz with you it's been confusion.

BAD MOM ARCHETYPE

Bad Mom Archetype: It was a projection of an introjection, not that I was angry at you man.

I had to accept the introjection to understand it wasn't me it was mom cuz I'm a sweet person.

Instead of thanking me for all the time she was here she was angry that she couldn't live here.

Lunatics thrive in lawless liberal cities. This triggers even more as our civilization ceases to be.

I know how far I can fall, I've been there before. Now I'm up, not taking any chances for sure.

Born clear we mal-adapt to a system awaiting us. Self-actualization occurs getting over this.

Self-actualization is individuation--becoming independent of systems--not doing something.

CONTAGIOUS MADNESS

Because the absence of these inlaid systems is clarity--how we were born: uniquely exalted energy.

What Sam Vaknin calls "nothingness" is what we want. Return to birth unencumbered and smart.

From clutter to clarity, it's like a lobotomy to be unencumbered with all those matrices.

As they mistreated [mis-identified] me I became far wimpier triggering more of the same see.

It's an unfair comparison saying you felt like a Jew in Nazi Germany but its the same syndrome see.

NOTHINGNESS: ON TOP OF WORLD

I'm on top of the world now but shudder looking back down the ladder as a naive seeker.

If you don't learn from your parents life will become a painful bootcamp til you don't take offense.

All my persecutors are dead now, it just seems like God takes em out. They were so arrogant.

Lived in a small desert town of liberals. You know how they hate conservatives, well it was hell.

Critics could break your windows and light your palm trees on fire, the cops would ignore it.

Once the culprits see they won't be arrested its like a trigger to torture victims to their death.

Life is magical now with miracles everywhere. That's how life is if undistracted by sin's lure.

Give into sin, become tunnel-visioned as miracles are shut out and over your head's a dark cloud.

CONTAGIOUS MADNESS

A habit persistently resisted will lose the drive for it. That wild desire is being fed giving into it.

SIN is a bad habit. We wish to supplant those brain grooves with good habits--routine/success.

REPENTANCE AND THE PINK CLOUD

Repentance brings a PINK cloud. It's not just the honeymoon period, it will persist to the end.

Sin more and it's the Fallen Hero Syndrome spiraling down. When you get up again, who knows?

To avoid bad memory we fall into our bag but the addiction only reinforces the memory dad.

Addiction is there to avoid something which only looms larger as the serpent spurs the addicting.

As I look out I see a beautiful crescent moon and streetlights. Before in sin, I saw only blight.

It's not who they are but demons they've accumulated somewhere. Encrustation of spirit: beware.

His wife knew he was seeing prostitutes cuz he'd start to look like a monster. Interesting to hear.

The greatest luxury to me is protection and safety. I feel so safe here after researching it thoroughly.

LETHAL MENTAL DISORDERS

There are isolating illnesses called Lethal Mental Disorders due to the suicides that follow.

If a mental illness causes death it's a Fatal Mental Illness and should be handled thusly: forgive thyself.

CONTAGIOUS MADNESS

Bulimia causes 18 times more suicides than other mental illnesses but this is about vanity you say?

I can digest one meal but not two. Learning your limitations is essential for success coming to you.

It is just now coming to light how bulimia is a fatal mental disorder based on shame/low self-worth.

If one recovers from bulimic behaviors but still has shame then he still needs therapy: it's chronic pain.

What they see as horrible and ugly--and it is--you've had to learn to live with, a withering invalid.

I have to remind myself daily: all those people are gone and won't be back, you've relocated in fact.

A lethal mental illness is where it's deadly and you still do it--what could be more obvious? Stop the dis

I think if a whole class of people are dying or don't make it past forty we oughta take a look at it: BULIMIA.

Bulimia is so deadly that most deaths happen while in the act. Think of that-- it is too horrible to fathom.

Bulimia is backed by Satan trying to kill that person via the most important thing for life: food.

THE DEMON IS AN UGLY GREEN THING

The bulimia demon is an ugly green thing and then everyone he knows comes against him.

To have mass starvation in WWII then this reversal in succeeding generations is global/historical.

It's the devil attaching to women's narcissism over the body, the KEY to their famished acceptance.

CONTAGIOUS MADNESS

The bulimic knows how ridiculous it all is so becomes more secretive until totally isolated or dead.

Bulimia abuse is twofold: [1] body-abuse having lasting results and [2] HATRED from everyone else.

Satan came to steal/kill/destroy and bulimia ends in death for attachment-traumatized girls and boys.

Since everyone HATES her she builds such a strong exterior battleship she becomes the best.

For who else but the attachment-traumatized would act like this, it is beyond ridiculous and hopeless.

THE RESULTS ARE GOOD *AND* BAD

It's good and bad. The bad was lost years of tears and the good is you now: a battle-hardened seer.

I must admit I always saw bulimia as a sin but now I see it as a possession attached to the heartbroken.

Food means MOTHER. Think of the far-ranging implications of that when she called you brat.

YOU'RE A PERSON NOT A DISEASE

Separate from anyone treating you as a disease not a person. You're recovering, take it easy friend.

It hurt so much being misjudged and then them acting like they owned me. It bloody shocked me actually.

Tho' my behavior brought on your meanness it gave me the opportunity to see you nevertheless.

My books are the only proof that I was here. I need you to know what I was thinking between my tears.

CONTAGIOUS MADNESS

Liberalism is thru all depts and women run em: education, churches, medicine and the list goes on.

The absence of bloat really makes a person stand out in the crowd. Imagine that, a cosmic joke so loud.

Music hits me on much deeper levels than boring politics. I'm gonna begin each morning with music.

CARNIVORE VS LOWFAT REVERSALS

The story of Daniel is good advice: he maintained youthful looks and vigor by living on wheat and water.

I am on a lowfat fruit/starch diet but I've been thru all of it and may even return to carnivore, who can predict it?

What to do with a skinny woman with wrinkled extremities: FAST HER and do it immediately.

Paul Bragg said Toxic Acid Crystals form in the extremities into the root. TAC is the basis for wrinkles too.

Like all tradition let your food-life be two-speed: regular daily routine vs. rare festival [if desired] meats.

TWO-SPEED FOOD LIFE

Thusly you have the beauty from non-acid foods and escape vitamineral or protein depletion if it exists.

Toxic acid crystals manifest in itchy dry wrinkles. It's all dried mucus [acid] under the skin gone in a day or so.

No more sauerkraut and spuds. Potatoes and tomatoes are becoming impossible as nightshades: acid reflux.

Instead of reflexively taking an ant-acid, investigate why you have it: to culture food you're horribly allergic.

CONTAGIOUS MADNESS

The simpler my diet to which I've adapted the more multi-variable I will be as a talented creative agent.

No more "natural cookies". Tho' made with coconut flour etc. they taste like dusty mildew/organisms creepy.

Make your own if you have a mind but I'd not get into all of that. Just eat one meal and lose your fat.

If you want all those deep wrinkles go eat all that food. It causes em, Berg's tables prove it's ACID/mucus.

How could we possibly need food that deforms the human body that way? It's so ugly it cannot be healthy.

I don't care if you drink or eat meat, have at it. I'm just talking about myself, it's personal not about all of ya.

Age doesn't have to deform you that way. There's no reason things should change, look at older Vietnamese.

The effects of culture food are so uglifying no artist could stand it and just to escape it would do anything.

CONTRADICTIONS AND REVERSALS

Like smearing oils and creams all over the dry wrinkled skin--it can all perfect but it's done from within.

When all the wrinkles left the body with a fruit diet everyone said I was gonna die from not eating meat.

That seemed to me a pathetic contradiction that the body could obviously heal, yet NOW it was ill?

That's the problem: I'm not a narcissist but I am an artist and I couldn't stand it, the deforming effects of ACID.

If hungry an orange cleans the gut of all elements incurring the pain. It doesn't take much--try a fig or date.

CONTAGIOUS MADNESS

Modern fruitarians didn't follow Ehret—he would never derail from fruit by stuffing with starches at night.

Don't listen to anyone. They'll say no nuts, no avocado, making you famished for everything ya' know.

A few nuts and avocado as your staff cuz you need the fat. Keep em ripening in refrigerator as your stash.

Let the cheese and dairy go for awhile. With just mucus-binding fruits lets see how you do: new style.

The fruitarian community became a dam Nazi tyranny and the forums were filled with arrogant meanies.

What food put me through: countless days/nights of acid reflux, burping, bloating but now I'm all new.

To escape them I became a vegetarian--including cheese. A French diet so to speak but still up a creek.

Roast a pig for your festival and pig-out on it. The rest of the time enjoy thy fruits/herbs to stay top notch.

OBSTRUCTIONS & THE CREATIVE ACT

Early rejection explains the insane drive for greatness and the survival panic leading to suicide.

Devil holds us back through remorse. Trigger-memories: anchors holding us down to the bad past.

Significance comes from identity of being a child of God and that gives you a purpose/not seen as odd.

The world imposes it's BS then weak friends get sucked in/create a mess and then they're high maintenance.

They don't want you to succeed. That needs to be focused on and wondered about, don't you agree?

CONTAGIOUS MADNESS

To succeed keep auditing your network for signs of friendship vs. frenemyshit. Are they even interested?

Do they create contention/division, are they predators of the heart, do they not want you to succeed?

AUDIT NETWORK

Audit Network: Do they hold you to the past and not want you to advance to your destiny and future?

Friendship is very rare/must be prized and held onto until you die. Problem is: world comes in, then bye bye.

The time is late, you've achieve something so great so now audit your network lest demons change your fate.

Do they want you to succeed? Or are they acting like a rudder bogging you down into the gutter?

Told to get along with her 1000 cousins of course she's validating sin in this era of porn and cruisin'.

It takes a long time to become young. Picasso

It wasn't just that. Things had been brewing under the surface and I just chose that event to wrap it up.

You got to cut em loose or you'll stay nothing, a caboose. They're not up to your par so fire em or lose.

Prosperity cannot be proof of God's favor since it's what Satan promises for those worshipping him.

All sins are attempts to fill voids. It's like a huge suction cup and in comes horrible things to avoid.

Imaginary evil is romantic and varied but real evil is monotonous, gloomy, barren and extremely boring.

IMAGINARY GOOD IS BORING

CONTAGIOUS MADNESS

Imaginary good is boring but real good always new, marvelous, relieving and intoxicating. S. Weil

Real good is the BEST--but kids don't see that, being sold a bunch of lies. Be good genius and open eyes.

You need a hobby or a true cause. not this weird extreme crap, it's deeply evil on the way to hell.

It was the devil you hated, not me. In weakness I bent and he overtook the vessel in my life's tragedy.

Driven by identity-panic cuz if I didn't work I wouldn't survive it: that's the history of all who made it.

Why bring up age? It's just abuse. I move and feel like I'm fifteen and work every waking minute too.

After you reject/fire the creep take a day to convalescence cuz you've felt damage with his mess.

Forgive: leave psychic space completely OPEN so God can fill it with ceaseless miracles one after another!

But the time is up for those who are corrupt.

I had to go through life in two stages: learning thru hurting (Ph.D. in the Streets) then success/reaping.

Stop cowering/sinking in your swill. These are all past tapes when you were overcoming and learning still.

The sinner should say: "I just want my intended life back."

It's horrifying what I'm finding out about em so more and more I'm succumbin' to my own cocoon.

Be smart you cute one you, don't read your reviews.

A MONUMENTAL ACHIEVEMENT: YOU

CONTAGIOUS MADNESS

It's the end of a long haul, a monumental achievement so now go slow, be deliberate, take it easy.

Don't fret you didn't follow your plan cuz it's all about God's plan, man! And that's what you've been doin'

Just because they find you unworthy of their attention you desperately want their attention more, man?

Don't resent past tyrants just see the system that brought it on: you were sick, addicted, negligent, down.

Feel as though I'll never get over it: Tyrants over me and kids invading me and I couldn't stand up to it.

It built certain muscles in me: constantly having to battle to get privacy, it ordered my life you see.

The Lord wanted me solo so he put me thru people-hell until I learned: lock the gate/end psychic smell.

How to complete a project: Lay out the frame, fill in the dots.

I'm off at noon, the Lord said He wanted receptivity--a switch from the tunnel vision of work obsession.

AS BODY RECEDES BRAIN EXPANDS

As the body recedes in old age the brain expands--imagine that.

Because I am maximally receptive the dark night of the soul was horrible, reading thoughts/no miracles.

I'm done, the ten world changing blockbusters are ready for ebook distribution or paperbacks if you choose.

Young love is about passion old love about accommodation--protecting the other's solitude in sun.

You're done with your work now it's just final touches, massage into perfection, deal with markets.

CONTAGIOUS MADNESS

Now done, turn your attention to another world. Release tunnel vision as you open up/avoid the lure.

I'm done with my work, it's locked into place. Now talking about the work: how man is disgraced.

Collaboration isn't always the key to success. More often they drag you down and the design's a mess.

PEOPLE ARE USUALLY JUST AN ENCUMBRANCE

He can't see, he doesn't remember me but he still loves Thee.

A rising tide rises all ships--I'll reward those helping. That's not me bragging I feel what's happening.

It's the complex human race in it's weird intricacies and devices to maintain homeostasis making us nuts.

Free willers scare me—they don't know the wonderful destiny God designed for free.

They don't search for the predestined groove we have with repentance, see?

Style to the end. Either you have it or you don't, friends

If you're an unread author what good are you?

This poetry came from deep emotions as I recall the lessons/never forget em.

Until it goes into production there are corrections! Now's not the time for complacency--focus!

Ten books and a billion details and it's all going into production and it's chaos and I love this.

To sell books ya gotta have the fame and you get that by goin' against the grain.

To feel really good look how far you've come. You're not done yet but man have you been accomplishin'.

CONTAGIOUS MADNESS

3/4 there--gonna go real slow to the finish line to make sure I didn't forget something/got the weekend.

COMPLETION!

Gonna party while I finish all weekend. Lookin' forward to the new life which will be opposite, yes ma'am.

You're 99.99% done but don't rush the finish, hon'! Handle like a crate of eggs, take the whole weekend.

Key to a masterpiece is patience. Never rush it just savor ride into completion and world success.

Hats off to my tech guy adapting to my extreme Harriet Craig attention to detail in this masterpiece.

You have reached a point in completion where even you can't muck it up.

You're done, hon'. It's just a matter of filling in the dots a bit more so today just party on/celebration

Oh come on, even he doesn't have all the answers. Stop this people worship and get back to nature.

Oh come on, even I don't have all the answers. Don't worship me or anyone else sir.

YOUR TIME WILL COME

Your time has come.

I'm done, my time has come and now we'll have fun after a long haul of decades overcoming dung.

She said I had delusions of grandeur. Please Lord, show her.

It took many decades but much of that was just suffering, learning and overcoming not writing.

Abnormal Psychology or Interactional Pathology (Systems Theory)?

CONTAGIOUS MADNESS

Once planting a seed instead of fearing "it" won't happen, get ready--for God said He would bless it, see?

I'm not gonna discuss my plans with you, why jinx em? You don't know what it is/what it took dumb dumb.

BE SMART ABOUT IT: STAY PRIVATE

The fastest way to ruin your life is discuss it with anyone so refuse to answer their insinuating questions!

You don't know anything about my life, what I do or what it's taken so shut fruitless questions/bye.

If someone has the truth they say it simply and if they don't they blab on falsely.

It's surival panic for a comic to engage people, coming from a neglectful mother and he'll do anything for it.

When you don't have a loving connection with the mother it's almost impossible to be disliked later.

Due to early rejection writers want world's approval 1000% and since that can't happen, die of alcoholism.

Steeped in resentments of dead long ago I am overwhelmed with survival panic fearing books unsold.

We're not at the end but the beginning of the end, the most important part so look up/savor it friends.

I never remembered your sins I just put you onto the next lessons. Lord

The decades of people-invasion weren't karma but lessons re: boundaries, wall/locked gate, assertion.

When you discipline children you hurt their feelings in the short term so they can act right in the future.

STYLE TO THE END OR YOU DON'T HAVE IT, FRIEND

CONTAGIOUS MADNESS

Style to the end, amen.

Stop cowering like a crushed person but forge ahead instead confident of God's power over walking dead.

Free willers come up with own thing but I'd rather find the groove the omniscient God designed for me.

Stop gauging self by likes. The mark of a true teacher is how many reject him for the truth so disliked.

Revel in minor problem solving at the end. The bumps in the road, savor em cuz it'll never happen again.

It was such a nightmare I went through but I had to go through it so I forgive all of it--I must to stay lit.

When I was younger I lacked the level of health I have now from high boundaries and staying hidden/low.

I just do what I do but what I went through to get here you wouldn't want to.

It's not that you're not finished. It's that you got such a huge handle on it--big chunk done re: increments.

You got the boulder up the hill, now it's just a few more mornings of tedious details so it's greater still.

Take a rest after getting that boulder up the hill. That way you're high as a kite when finally there/thrilled.

JUST BE NICE: CORDIAL BUT "WARM STEEL"

Mediation tends to soften people's entrenched positions.

I only have confidence in myself, doing what I gotta do to get around em but expecting nothing from em.

I got the boulder up the hill and perfectly finished last minute details. I'm done, thriving, prepared, no fail.

CONTAGIOUS MADNESS

Gotta know who you are to be a star. Avoid ego--it's Who's you are, all glory goes to God the Father.

I don't care how much of % they get of my work as long as they make me rich, my penury is the gist.

Finished the last details and now really done. How anticlimactic though, nothing is happenin'.

When I track mind into what they have to say--and altho' it's interesting and ok--it's less than my reality.

FALL OUT OF STRUCTURE

Constantly un-track the mind, coming into your own moment where past and future unite in new notions.

With all that work behind me I just wanna retire into the fat moment by desk-clearing and seeking clarity.

Retirement is enlightenment from falling out of structure: that tiresome tracking not the mind of the Lord.

I hereby transcend all political psychology (current events) in favor of my own reality and future suspense.

It's not eldering "work", it's eldering consciousness--sagacity--where you return to childhood, free.

Everything was so great in my childhood! Our world splintered in the sixties and we all lost our sanity.

Tho' TV is good it's always lower. Same with videos, other views, people in news, whatever--I'm higher.

A big balloon is my symbol of freedom: flying away from the work done, reveling in great achievement won.

SEE THE SIGNS: MIXED SIGNALS OF THE SLIME

CONTAGIOUS MADNESS

The reason we don't talk is I'll never give you a chance to hurt me again chump.

I know how fast all can fail so I got humility and solid dependence on God: for success set sail.

From a cold heart/seared conscience you're young again, pliable in God's hands, nice but sly as fox.

Let music be your default setting. Always return to calmness, expansive thoughts, confident/happy.

Desire for approval for what you're achieved is a natural and worthwhile goal for in God it was conceived.

Don't worry they get it from what you've already presented--it's done, you've won, retirement is fun.

I'm happy with my quality of life now and more money won't change that-- it's good to know it.

As one becomes a success the others reject those who haven't made it yet and the result: mental illness.

When the successful one is also evil, the whole clan becomes dispossessed if they worship moneyed people.

When the weasel becomes the king and the superior man remains on the periphery: hell to pay.

I've studied genius and saints all my life. I'm not saying I'm one but there is a hierarchy liberals deny.

I'm always more interested in working than marketing so I ran outa money and there was little/no selling.

LEAVE A LEGACY THROUGH STRICT ROUTINE

Now I've grown up and am reviving all this. I'm leaving a legacy I confess.

Strict routine office hours: Office One, am-noon (with dogs). Office Two: noon-5 pm (with cats to love).

CONTAGIOUS MADNESS

It's the end of a long haul, a monumental achievement so now go slow, be deliberate, take it easy.

Don't fret you didn't follow your plan cuz it's all about God's plan, man! And that's what you've been doin'

Just because they find you unworthy of their attention you desperately want their attention more, amen?

COOL REJECTIONS WAKE YOU UP

Their cool rejection was the ontologically fatal insight preceding psychotic shock from a family who sucked.

Don't resent past tyrants just see the system that brought it on: you were sick, addicted, negligent, down.

In other words, don't sink in your swill.

You have every right to be proud of yourself for all you've accomplished. SEE this by taking distance!

Six books and 8 long picturestrips to be viewed and enjoyed while you vaca and live off results of your toil.

I did the best I know how, and I was driven. Though fired by neurosis/need for attention I did it/I'm retirin'

Not just need for justified recognition but driven to know my Self and all God had been pre-designin'

I can see it happening---a giant deja-vu. I knew it in my mind's eye--always working towards it, whew!

Anyone can look you up, that's the point. So just make your books available then wait/have a joint.

I want it all behind me though, the intense focus/work load. I want to open up, take distance, relax ya know?

CREATIVE ACT IS A STRUCTURE IN NATURE!

CONTAGIOUS MADNESS

In all fields it's the same thing and process. Seed, germination, completion: had a guess/overcame mess.

Tho' all they did was try your patience, reward people for trying. With poor character though, fire em.

Let it occur while you detour: the explosion from your work. You were sent by God, it fits this era perf.

You worked but also waited--you were patient, man! Not many worthless accomplishments but One.

What a thrill it is to be done, as completion is part of nature! I'm exalted as my eyes go to the future.

You planted a helluva seed, I'm mean it's huge. Now just wait for the inevitable to occur and get ready too.

It's all gonna happen just like you always thought. You had a lifelong vision and it was God you sought.

I love to think futuristically--outa the present box, to be free: fantastic productivity and money.

No matter how good it is it's lower than my own reality so why bother, just proceed so they're freed.

Your own personal reality is hard-won because it means overcoming the scum of social hypnotism.

Exhausted scientist said "Now I'm old, now it's happening but that's the way things go undoubtedly."

THE DEN OF LASCIVIOUS LIBERALISM

Those who hate the truth call truth "hate".

I judged myself through their eyes. They saw me as insignificant, replaceable, not worth a cent.

It's not science it's a fad, and mental illness is not a civil right.

CONTAGIOUS MADNESS

Not just Obama but an entire generation who supported him. He was smooth and they were lulled.

The nitpicking and scrutinizing for offense is now getting much more intense.

Culture is falling into chaos and debauchery like old civilizations in bible filled with monsters and murder.

Be careful of "gay Christians" or "gay conservatives" cuz they are activists when it comes to their "issue".

HAVE IMMUNITY AGAINST TYRANNY

The second amendment is our immune system against tyranny so that is why we defend it like crazy.

Unhinged, deranged leftists driven to insanity by a lying left-wing media feeding the frenzy on a daily basis.

Not "news" but smearing innocent people while encouraging mass hysteria and violence in left-wing lunatics.

Media driving America into a bloody civil war in their desperate attempt to destabilize the nation.

Let's get em shooting in the streets then call in UN "peacekeeping" troops, depose Trump, disarm pop.

No more public speaking if you can't monitor the crowd. In the good ol' days people were decent/mild.

Conservatives must start thinking about security. Never go to restaurants or places without it, surely!

The kids are told "everything fun in life is illegal, immoral or fattening". So do whatever you want Kathy.

DISCOVER WHAT YOUR KIDS ARE TAUGHT!

Discover what your child is being taught (and groomed for) to accept as "normal, good and natural."

CONTAGIOUS MADNESS

Dems desperate Kavanaugh will tip the balance so they can't kill babies anymore and thus their tactics.

The cold dems wanna maintain sexual irresponsibility by killing babies when it comes to Roe vs. Wade.

Gang rape allegations: If this is how the dems act outa power how would they act in/with Hillary Clinton?

The huge gay lobby is constantly ranking the corporations/upping their criteria to avoid prosecution.

Gay lobby long tendrils: They'll monitor a company's gay standards but also those of their vendors.

They're always building the frame of the argument and we're always reacting to the frame and feel framed.

They cut all videos of ex-gays because they "demean homosexuality". The only way out is Jesus, truthfully.

Someone once said "If sodomy's not wrong, nothing's wrong."

America cannot be exceptional if it promotes and celebrates the advancement of the homosexual sin.

Moderates like Dana Perino are socially liberal republicans/increasingly going along with the gay plan.

These liberal moderates are openly trying to make the republican party pro-homosexual like it's swell.

Growing LBGT tyranny is swallowing us/every institution up like quicksand or a cobweb/we're sick of em.

In the name of non-discrimination, they discriminate. In the name of civil rights, they take away rights.

SIN IS NEVER SYNCHRONICITY (RIGHT SIDE OF HISTORY)

CONTAGIOUS MADNESS

Sin is never on the "right side of history" because it transgresses the design of the Creator of it all, God.

They can't fill desires with God so there's a restlessness there and perversions are always expanding.

They're nurturing homosexual identity and since behavior flows from identity they do bathhouses/disgusting.

Left: performance anger, destruction theatre or inciting violence against those who hate their behavior.

This isn't a war with a front you can see, but a bunch of weasels and losers sniping behind the scene.

End Transgender Tyranny.

Estrogen turns the man into a handicapped man and the testosterone in the woman to a handicapped man.

Oppose transgender child abuse.

People for traditional values have become second class citizens under the law as they hammer in anti-God.

The Sexual Revolution is a totalitarian ideology--it relies on force. It's not for Christians of course.

The church needs to help homosexuals but not concede and cave in to gay activists/let their stuff in.

Grotesque/well-coordinated character assassination by democrats and "Dr. Ford" raised a mil to pay for it.

Geo Soros sends 246 million to pro-abortion groups to smear Kavanaugh. Thought he was behind it.

LIBERALS SAY WE'RE ALL REPLACEABLE

When liberals replace you easily the message is you're not worthy and if you're not sure of yourself, bye bye.

CONTAGIOUS MADNESS

Their cool rejection was the ontologically fatal insight preceding psychotic shock from a family who sucked.

Confusion: We were always told racism is of the far right but now liberals are loudest against whites.

We're entering most prosperous times in America and it makes the Trump haters even more enraged at ya.

Liberals used to say don't judge by skin color but now it's all they do as they try to aggravate a race war.

Love can only beat terrorism if it has lots of guns. Would it have worked with Hitler? Of course not hon'.

Main shovedown since kindergarden: "We're all one" and it's B.S. hon'!

Lack of rationality is too much for me. Calling anyone who thinks differently a racist and they believe it.

THE PAST IS A LESSON THAT'S ALL

Feeling of being censured and misjudged is so breathtakingly appalling it's not worth it staying in the ring.

They are so creepy as through social hypnotism they believe what they're saying and it's frightenin'

The more progressive ideologue Millennials take over the more I just wanna get away/the heck outa here...

There's a callousness to you guys. You think you're not callous but you're the most callous of all.

It's just too eerie being banned, censored and scorned. This isn't America it's a progressive hell adorned.

Don't shudder as thou looks back. It was wisdom from age you lacked when you had the herd's back.

CONTAGIOUS MADNESS

You literally didn't know what you were doing. That's what Lord said as demons blinded/made us lowly.

When liberals replace you easily the message is you're not worthy and if you're not sure of yourself, bye bye.

Simply put: The reason we love him is the reason they hate him. That's how wide the gulf is again.

Because they follow the narrative not bible they just mumble and stutter trying to explain their behavior.

Yes you were a sinner and that's why they turned on you but it gave you a view of their utter badness too.

The bible is the central document of western culture, defining truth and how we should act (mature).

Inequality of Outcome is always blamed on patriarchy or whitiies. Never IQ, the reason for discrepancy.

MASSIVE IMMIGRATION IS DESTRUCTIVE SAVAGERY

Obama was pro-war yet--unbelievably--all anti-war protests from the left stopped/wanted power more.

Obama spent 1.6 million restoring graffiti of communist dictators. Che Guevara, Castro and other traitors.

Obama tried to outlaw family farms, raising the demand for illegal immigrants (we were alarmed).

Since most criminals are black, Obama said it's racial discrimination to not hire criminals, imagine that.

Under Obama Americans on food stamps went from 33 to 49 million, beginning the homeless problem.

They don't want massive immigration cuz they love em but to change society by destructive savagery.

CONTAGIOUS MADNESS

People don't hate immigrants they don't want their society to change--our traditions/bible, deranged.

Hillary, Barrack and Megan all grandstanded using a tragedy to put their own agenda out—we're disgusted.

Democrats will always use a crisis to grandstand, ever taking advantage of the opportunity but a funeral? Really...

Just like Italians suddenly reversed against Mussolini, it's happening suddenly against Obama, the creep.

And we're sick of all the gratuitous sex on TV too.

Hollywood awards viewers down 20% last year. We're sick of the hatred and Trump smears.

They're mad Donald was golfing during funeral but he was not invited, so what do they expect, ya know?

Bowed his head to Jesus, He stood for Uncle Sam, he only loved one woman and proud of all he had.

Our sweet life suddenly changed thru regulation. We feared a knock at the door, a police state nation.

The eight years of hell Hussein Obama brought on us: The police state, the fears, the frustrations.

Truth only comes from unbridled speech. Straight from the cuff, fearless, shameless, guilt-free.

THE CHURCHES HAVE FALLEN

Most churches are forsaken, cum-baya, false doctrine, filled with demons/no bible.

I came from a blue state. When I realized it was liberalism creating treachery and hate, I escaped.

Believe in somethin'--even if it's a lie, believe in it! Colin Kaepernick

CONTAGIOUS MADNESS

Everybody and their mama having babies outa wedlock and the preacher don't say nothin' about it.

Equality is a dangerous myth.

Civilized restraint is the antidote to chaos.

Who is supercilious? The leftists. We as conservatives just wanna be left alone and we're serious.

They pour out arrogant words, speaking hard things: all the evildoers boast loftily. Jude 14, 15

LGBT Agenda snuck into "Character Education".

School book "Marked" describes having sex in the hallways or with students, now common incidents.

Fallen false preacher going along with LGBT agenda: "I would rather err on the side of love, not truth."

They want you to look the other way so that they can do as they see fit with you and your children.

I'm not against pronouns I'm against legislation about what words I can utter.

The gender pronouns required are artificial constructions of radical ideologues whom I do not respect.

When you have to start hiding things to publish or renaming it to prevent possible offense.

"KINDNESS" IS ALWAYS THE EXCUSE

Kindness is always the excuse when the SJW's wanna control what people think, say, do and support.

The highest value is TRUTH not "kindness".

Kindness means supporting perverts.

CONTAGIOUS MADNESS

SJW's aren't motivated by "kindness" but power.

As a result of Obama's hustling white people are hated more today than anytime in the world's history.

Police officers are under attack more today than anytime in American history due to Obama's treachery.

Undermining our alliances, cozying up to Russia--what happened to our republican party? --Obama

Reps aren't cozying up to the KGB, it's just more lies. "If you want your doctor you can keep him"—all disguise.

If you wouldn't make a speech like that in the 1950s with dirty words, you shouldn't do it now sir.

WHAT I WROTE WHEN EATING MEAT

Are we Obligate Carnivores? Carnivores eat fruit and leaves. It's a matter of proportion, which varies.

Carnivores eat fruit and leaves. Even if a little lemon on their fish, it's fruit and I love yogurt with berries.

When I finally ate meat after decades of rabbit food my whole world opened up in a colorful phantasmagoria.

Flesh is not a dirty thing but what we're supposed to eat. I may not like it either but truthfully I sure feel great.

I'm satisfied from next to nothing cuz it's the right thing: Morning cream and berries, meat for brunch, fast.

The onslaught from ex-veganism is ruthless and vicious so you must now man-up to enjoy the delicious.

It's funny how everything is opposite: Meat-eaters have stable moods/are peaceful, not the rabbit-fooders.

CONTAGIOUS MADNESS

I noticed meat-eating men looked very handsome like the carnivorous actors from way back when.

It's totally enjoyable switching from meat to fruit and back again. They are a perfect balance to maintain.

Marinate your meats with fruits like berries. It's meat and fruits that go together and rabbits eat the veggies.

Two grapes and I was full, satisfied. You don't have to eat truckloads like they say, just balance/even pies.

Balance: Eat fruit then balance with meat. Fast, then balance again and it's all instructed by your system.

Many vegans are so deficient they dream of pot roast every night. A very dangerous thing/a blight.

MacDougal reasons: since all continents exist on starch it must be right. That's typical liberal science, hah.

HANDSOME AND PRETTY 1950'S

In the fifties when people were handsome and pretty this woulda been a no-brainer: meat on the platter.

Now they make concoctions to replace meat and it's sickening, we won't even touch these man-made things.

Green powders stuck in liver: When ex-vegans take colonics to rid the past it's a a green snake they eject.

The future will laugh at this era when people bought pills, powders and potions and we all spent a fortune.

I'm so enjoying my breakfast: sour cream with berries, I'm high as a kite/merry.

Don't discuss your diet cuz they all come down on you for it since there's always two sides so forget it.

CONTAGIOUS MADNESS

Every plant and animal has self-defense--veggies don't wanna be eaten! That's why I get sick and hate em.

Fruits are ok but I prefer FATS. Animal fat (fauna) keeps my brain in tune, high energy, focus and gladness.

To think I tried to get the fat from avocado or nuts! How useless, I go right to the source of confusion.

Go ahead and stay on plant diet while I live life to it's fullest and am what I am cuz I eat what God gave us.

Gave my dogs raw beef yesterday--they ate it up so happily, now I see why they won't eat cooked meat.

Put one pineapple chunk in my raw milk shake with yogurt. There, I had my fruit and I'm better for it.

Carnivores eat fruit and leaves. It's a matter of proportion which varies but right now via meat I'm sweet.

Keep veggies for rabbits cuz for humans they're filled with anti-nutrients--what a laugh since the 60's.

NOW: A VERY SMALL SHOPPING LIST

In the Old West they went to town once a month to get butter, bacon and coffee.

It used to be the roast was the main dish but now if you bring it you're seen as a murdering creep/accomplice.

All wrinkles leave body suddenly since it's same bloodstream running thru every cell/thank you daddy.

What is a feast? Something magnificent which allows you to fast 2-3 days afterwards at least.

After learning all about diets you ultimately have to be your own guru and then shut up about it.

CONTAGIOUS MADNESS

With animal foods/no starch or sugar I experienced a Maxfield Parrish reality of castles and fairytales.

Animal foods diet means daily fasting cuz the satiety is implied: how lil' ladies stayed skinny in the fifties.

Ex-vegans attacked by vegans the same way liberals attack anyone who escapes their grip, how sick.

After resuming meat after decades: everything worked perfectly and that horrible dry skin went away.

Durianrider and Freelee reeled me back so many times, they're good salesmen of veganism I'll say that.

It was always the animal cruelty issue that made me drop new heath to truckle back in and avoid the feud.

After meat: Wow! So THIS is how I'm supposed to feel--the way I did as a kid, before the shovedown pill.

It was beautiful people of the 50's-60's and it was stolen from them with margarine/lowfat doctrine.

WOW! THIS IS HOW I'M SUPPOSED TO FEEL!

I thought: Wow! So this is how I'm supposed to feel--the way I did as a kid, before this false fix.

The beautiful people of the 50's-60's and it was stolen from them with margarine and lowfat doctrine.

It was always the animal cruelty issue that made me drop new heath to truckle back in and avoid the feud.

Low fat vegan dogma (shove down) hurt dogs too. They were deprived of table leavings/delicious food.

It's a food paradox: fruit makes ya bitchy as hell and meat makes you (again) a sweet little boy or girl.

CONTAGIOUS MADNESS

When fat melted off and I got my synapses back, Wow: electricity running thru cholesterol is perfect.

I often switch from lowcarb to paleo all cuz I wanna eat fruit.

On vegetable oils like olive I had belly fat but when I substituted with animal fat it ALL went away.

Ate a pear and thought I'd die for a day. Gut ache: meat digests sooo smoothly and fiber is self-hate.

This comes from the severe digestive disorders resulting from veganism which has never occurred on earth.

Broccoli isn't even a real vegetable and many veggies poison eaters for protection/avoid em man.

Everything comes down to synapses and all wiring is insulated in fat which means lowfat diets = insanity.

LACK OF ANIMAL FAT = INSANE (MENTALLY FLAT)

I was insane for decades from the lack of animal fat. Avocados didn't do it, olive oil nothing to it.

The irrational fear of meat--did you have it as a kid? No, we took it all for granted then, it was IT.

I felt like crap with all that fiber in the gut. With meat I'm so stable/smooth/sleek with high energy/strut.

Insulation for all wiring in us is cholesterol and that's the very thing they told us to avoid? Incredible

I don't like it any more than you do but I gotta do it to survive cuz, I'm sick with fiber, starch, sugar/no jive.

Ex-vegan carnivores eat meat and organs raw. Sorry I can't do that for it's enough just to eat it at all.

CONTAGIOUS MADNESS

Lowfat = Weak control over actions/words as autonomisms (uprushes from the unconscious) occurred.

Finally, we don't have to fear vegan's reactions to our new direction pursuing wellness despite the angry.

I wasn't myself and could never be myself cuz that's based on animal fat which I cut out, just like that.

Eating meat even has to do with family bonding. They meet to eat, very important and warmin'

Anti-nutrients: That's what veggies have and I'm thinking of my uncle who refused em/only ate bread.

Since I gave up fiber I feel so much better. The gut unblocked from matter made me visibly fitter.

If you can't eat meat or non-fruit find one protein you can, regain your immunity then you can eat it all.

Haven't tried raw eggs/liver/heart yet but promise I'll get to it.

VEGAN CABAL IS LIBERAL & NEW WORLD ORDER

Vegans are part of liberal cabal as well as NWO. Those who don't get sucked in maintain health in gold.

Even a little fiber and I have a truck in my gut. Obligate carnivores are fit/flat with all belly fat out.

They portray the anti-nutrients in plants and even soy as "healthy". They always do that and thus we die.

Over 80% of vegans/vegetarians go back to eating meat. Why, if it's so great and perfect for the peeps?

Bill Gates supports depopulation--and fake meat. Hmmm

Fake meat, NWO veganism = zombie apocalypse. Heck, can't you see it in their eyes as we speak?

CONTAGIOUS MADNESS

Though it looks like a healthy trend veganism is actually Satanic. Hitler did it, heavy metal bands do it.

Hollywood is very into it, you hear about it everywhere. NWO brainwash, like Ellen eats her carrots.

I will not be surprised when all the liberal (FALSE) churches go vegan. Even now church sites are joining in.

Very prevalent now: Churches giving diet advice and vegan is in. They see it as holy/more virtue signalin'

Churches will be serving fake meats at their potlucks and no one would think of bringing a pot roast.

Used to be the guest bringing the beef roast was a real hero but not he'd be embarrassed to.

VEGANS LOST THEIR TEETH

Ex-vegans all lost their teeth and now eat nothing but meat. They can't digest the rest/made em effete.

Just as the water reflects the stars and the moon, the body reflects the mind and soul. Rumi quotes

The Walmart pie said "freshness guaranteed" as it stood fresh on the shelf for one year/don't believe.

When you eat, eat the most calorically dense possible--not rabbit food. Cowboy Levoy Finicum

My interest in daily fasting is not anorexia but a spiritual calling. Like some are called to celibacy, it's my thing.

With the wrong premise people lose their intelligence and they'll all see it when things don't add up.

ROAST at 375 for 3 hours: Cut tomatoes tossed with olive oil, salt, pepper and lotsa garlic--enjoy it.

CONTAGIOUS MADNESS

Vegans say "no oil" but that's bull if you're in for the long haul. Potato chips: sliced/ S&P/olive oil, broil.

I learned at 15 I didn't have normal digestive apparatus with only one possible digestive burn a day.

I just wanna appreciate this day, a Saturday. I haven't eaten yet, why spoil it--not hungry just wanna think.

Vegans are like all SJW's--rude and cruel as they hammer in the speel of the cool tyrannizing over you.

Restore old paths and 18" waists.

Lberal (vegan) persecution for eating meat is so violent and opprobrious most can't recover their health.

Many gurus of raw veganism admit to eating cooked food, ice cream or animal products--yet are selling this.

POOR DECISIONS OF VEGANS

As a vegan I made poor decisions making me sicker then seeking of superfoods and snake oil potions etc.

Vegans also promote vasectomies--stripping you of a future family and that is a cruel horrible tragedy.

And to think family complained of "hunger for something" and instead of giving em meat I gave em a seed.

I experimented with Daily Fasting Eating Anything for years to prove a point but now I want what's right.

Dogs are so happy with pot roast aromas going thru the house. They too see veganism as ridiculous.

Happy cute meat-eating kid. Met a man who called me unkind so I went vegan and lost health and mind.

CONTAGIOUS MADNESS

Twenty years: acid burn as vegan. Thought I had esophageal cancer hon' but as an ex-vegan pain is gone.

As vegan I was so dizzy I often had to sit down. I lost immunity, every chemical affected me, frown.

Losing teeth, often angry, aging early and dry skin: that's the vegan and I'm sorry to pop your vision.

It's not ugly aging is from not eating meat. It's living on non-nutritive starches and sweet fruits/effete.

Vegan trip was part of liberalism and the globalist's plan to bring us down. Deficiencies of effete, overrun.

Proclamation: Forcing vegan dogma on cats and dogs is cruel and wrong!

The cruelty thing took over minds and we saw meat-eaters as evil and meat itself as dirty/despicable.

Vegans look great at first but as reserves are depleted and deficiencies rear up they fail to thrive/I lived it.

VEGAM DOCTORS: NO CREDENTIALS JUST CREDO

The vegan doctors had no credentials they just believe the credo, a mouthful.

Like a giant conspiracy: Lure us to accept dogma making us sick so we buy your snake oil tricks.

No bigger clash: traditional meat eating family with a new vegan justice warrior looking like a horror.

When I went vegan at 22 I instantly developed an eating disorder but couldn't see it like Karen Carpenter.

Give em what they want/are hungry for: meat. Nothing else satisfies, seems nutritious or doesn't exist.

Why are patients given plant-based diet? To keep em in the system so there's no recovery to fight it.

CONTAGIOUS MADNESS

Wanting meat so bad but not able to go against orthorexic dogma inside. Extremely dangerous/I tried it.

I would not eat the dirty thing--meat. The cruelty. So for years--decades--I continued but I'm back.

I feel so much better three days into the paleo-fast. Wow, wow, wow after years of hazy fatigue in the past.

Stop forcing your poor dogs and even cats to eat cauliflower you cruel creepy vegan monsters.

I hate to say it, I really do: but all the basic nutrients are in the meat not the plants and I'm sorry for you.

After years of confusion I'm filled with energy as an obligate carnivore which means fasting more.

Meat: After years of 10-banana smoothies etc. I have clarity/energy and what a lesson for America.

LOWFAT DOGMA UGLY AND DUMB?

Ladies were beautiful/gents handsome but then in came low fat dogma and they became ugly/dumb.

All were thin/good-looking but then TV ads said "no butter--just margarine" and we all succumbed.

To see an entire culture go from beauty and brains to dumb squares in pain is so telling/instructive, just sayin'

Many scientists knew it too: the way to bring down the west was to make em sick as hell and depressed.

Low-fat vegan so messed up my health now all I can eat is meat/zero-carb which reversed defeat.

Ruined metabolism thru lowfat vegan means you're now an obligate carnivore/ageless star.

CONTAGIOUS MADNESS

The obligate carnivore sees disappearance of wrinkles, dry skin, baseless fears or nothing happenin'

Angelina Jolie--a world beauty--has bacon and eggs every morning then nothing, you see?

As a tired vegan I got addicted to caffein pills and ruined my health even more. Now not--energy galore!

Vegans are lousy workers. Being brain fogged/fuzzy they start to take superfoods and powders.

Powders, pills and potions don't work. They stay in the liver, a big slimy green ball making tiredness worse.

After losing my teeth from fruit-only diet I was still so utopian-brainfogged I argued with the dentist.

A happy meat eater as a teen, when I switched to vegan it was the worst eating disorder ever seen.

MEAT MADE US HUMAN *AND* HUMANE

You take away a person's sustenance--the thing making him human and his True Self--and it's hell.

What I went through for decades of mental illness and skinny fat unfitness was one for the Guinness.

What I went thru with the inability to handle people, the lack of boundaries and assertion against invaders/evil.

Just like an alcoholic goes to lowlife. it was the same with lost destiny from rejecting what I needed for life.

You can't develop musculature on anything but meat. Those vegan body builders are a scam, believe me.

Genius and saints are pure, kind to animals but that doesn't mean they are vegan--that's new age/false.

CONTAGIOUS MADNESS

Switch from lowcarb to paleo when you wanna eat fruit.

Forget avocado, coconut, olive oil--it doesn't work for dry skin. Use butter baby, the real thin'

While writing of cornucopia I had no sense of it cuz I wasn't eating meat--it was illusion: child's view of utopia.

On the first meat day my whole life opened up and it was true cornucopia, vivid perception, lucid recall.

Here I was, an obligate carnivore due to low immunity and I removed my only lifeline due to virtue signaling.

Here I was, a sweet meat-eating child with huge potential who bought the trip that veganism was essential.

A CUTE KID BECOMES A VEGAN BIGOT

I became a ovo-lacto-rasta vegetarian but I'm afraid that wasn't enough. It's in the red meat, liver and blood.

The very things we needed to be handsome blueprints of humans and they said drop this dangerous vermin.

Stop forcing your poor dogs and even cats to eat cauliflower you cruel creepy vegan monsters.

The whole point of the meat is I don't have to eat again, see? But it's where the minerals are they tell me.

Low fat vegan dogma (shove down) hurt dogs too. They were deprived of table leavings/delicious food.

It's a food paradox: fruit makes ya bitchy as hell and meat makes you (again) a sweet little boy or girl.

When fat melted off and I got my synapses back, wow: electricity running thru cholesterol is perfect.

P.S. Carnivores also eat fruit.

CONTAGIOUS MADNESS

As you get clear from right foods you realize how many have victimized you in your lowered state--whew!

Use the starches **BEANS/RICE/CORN/SPUDS** for your staff of life. They're how man has lived from the beginning.

WHEN A FAT-FRUITARIAN

Food Today: Three red grapefruits, one small avocado, three mangos, tab. almond butter, half coconut.

Get frozen fruits and fill several freezers. That's for smoothies then add coconut, superherbs and nutbutters.

The closest I get to a salad is cilantro in my guacamole and also tomato, green onion, garlic, lemon.

I just drink my guacamole green goddess breakfast as a pudding then I'm done: fruit, greens, fat.